Living with Hepatitis C For Dummies

Hepatitis C Do's and Don'ts

Living well with hepatitis C is possible! Here are some suggestions based on three simple ideas: Take good care of yourself, communicate with your doctor, and learn about hepatitis C and how to treat it.

- ✔ Drink plenty of water. Your cells are mostly made of water and need regular filling up after water is lost by breathing, urinating, and sweating.

- ✔ Get enough rest. Sleep well at night and take naps if you need them (earlier in the day if possible).

- ✔ Reduce stress. Try proper breathing techniques, meditation, Yoga, and T'ai Chi.

- ✔ _____ larly. Try walking, stretching, swimming, or cycling.

- ✔ E_____ not hungry, eat small nutritious meals thro_____ day.

- ✔ Get support. Turn to your family, friends, and support groups for help.

- ✔ Find a liver specialist. Find and regularly visit a physician who has experience in treating hepatitis C

- ✔ Do keep all your medical papers together. Write down questions and concerns for your doctor and find one place to store all the paperwork.

- ✔ Tell your doctor about any changes in your symptoms. He may want to order some tests or alter your medication.

- ✔ Read *Living with Hepatitis C For Dummies.* Become informed about the virus, how it affects you, and what you can do about it.

Along with the things to do are the things you shouldn't do:

- ✔ Don't drink alcohol. Alcohol use can further damage your liver.

- ✔ Don't smoke. Chemicals in cigarettes are toxic.

- ✔ Don't use street drugs. Injection drug use is the major route of hepatitis C infection, as well as other infections.

- ✔ Don't stop your interferon or ribavirin medication. If you're having trouble with your medication, call your doctor first.

- ✔ Don't use any new medications or herbs without discussing them with your doctor first. Many over-the-counter products, prescription medicines, and herbal remedies can hurt your liver.

- ✔ Don't give up hope! A positive outlook can be your most powerful tool in fighting this illness.

Living with Hepatitis C For Dummies®

Protecting Others from Infection

Hepatitis C is transmitted via blood, so to keep others safe, just be careful with anything that may have your blood on it, as in the following examples:

- Keep any household object or item that may have your blood on it (such as razors and toothbrushes) safely away from others, especially children.

- Keep your wounds covered. Carry bandages with you in your car, wallet, or purse.

- Carefully wrap up and dispose of any items that may have blood from menstruation or a wound.

- Inform your sex partners about your hepatitis C. If you have multiple or new partners or practice sex with exposure to blood, use a latex barrier (condom or dental dam).

- Don't share any drug paraphernalia at all if you inject or snort drugs.

- Don't donate organs or give blood.

Tips for Partners of Folks with Hepatitis C

Because hepatitis C is usually a long-term chronic illness, you have lots of opportunities to help your loved one through his or her challenges.

- **Inform yourself about hepatitis C:** Find out about hepatitis C virus transmission, the disease, and treatment. Reading this book will give you lots of information.

- **Be positive:** If you aim to be supportive rather than critical, you have a better chance of helping your mate.

- **Develop a healthy lifestyle:** Change your diet, give up cigarettes, start walking, and do it together!

- **Provide practical help:** It's the day-to-day things that matter, like going along to the doctor's office, doing a little extra around the house, and helping with health care paperwork.

Copyright © 2005 Wiley Publishing, Inc. All rights reserved.

Item 7620-8.

For more information about Wiley Publishing, call 1-800-762-2974.

For Dummies: Bestselling Book Series for Beginners

Living with Hepatitis C

FOR

DUMMIES®

by Nina L. Paul, PhD

Foreword by Gina Pollichino, RN

WILEY

Wiley Publishing, Inc.

Living with Hepatitis C For Dummies®

Published by
Wiley Publishing, Inc.
111 River St.
Hoboken, NJ 07030-5774
www.wiley.com

WILEY

About the Author

Nina L. Paul, PhD, has worked in the field of science and health communication for 22 years. She started down this path at SUNY Purchase, where she received her bachelor's degree in biology and performed research in the field of neuroimmunology.

After working in medical publishing at Rockefeller University Press *(Journal of Clinical Investigation),* she received her master's degree and PhD in infectious disease epidemiology and immunology from Yale University.

After leaving Yale, Nina pursued postdoctoral research in England. Nina's research focused on human immunodeficiency virus (HIV) and related viruses and their interaction with the immune system. As part of her research, she published research articles and presented her results at scientific conferences around the world.

Nina also taught science to schoolchildren in New Mexico and volunteered at a hospital-based Cancer Information Centre in England. She worked in the field of evidence-based medicine and contributed to the Cochrane Library (a medical database).

Nina believes in a multifaceted approach to health. She became a master of reiki, which is a universal life-force energy that is transmitted through the hands. Check out Nina's Web site at www.ninapaul.info.

Dedication

I dedicate this book to my mother, Harriet Paul.

Author's Acknowledgments

Here is the place where I thank the "village" that helped me to write this book.

I'm grateful for the support of loving family and friends: the Paul clan — Marvin (my father), David, and Joshua; The Kasmanoff's — Caryn, Sam, Nathan, Noah, and Anna; The Sularski's — Suzette, Allan, and Rebecca; Thelea Fudim, Bunny Kunin, and Henry Gotthelf; the four Barbaras, Annette, Sue, Patti, Cindy, Robin, Lily, Gus, and Burton, and all my other friends and Reiki angels.

I thank the editorial team, including Natasha Graf, who came up with the idea for this book and brought me to it; Mike Baker, who contributed valuable experience and perspective as project editor; Tina Sims, copyeditor, who has the sharpest eyes; and George Nikias, MD, who heads a hepatitis C clinic in New Jersey and served as technical editor.

An angel brought Gina Pollichino, RN, who has shared her enthusiasm and knowledge about hepatitis C and wrote the foreword to this book.

To the people living with hepatitis C, their family and friends, and their doctors who have shared their stories with me, a huge thank you.

Publisher's Acknowledgments

We're proud of this book; please send us your comments through our Dummies online registration form located at www.dummies.com/register/.

Some of the people who helped bring this book to market include the following:

Acquisitions, Editorial, and Media Development

Project Editor: Mike Baker

Acquisitions Editors: Natasha Graf, Mikal Belicove

Senior Copy Editor: Tina Sims

Editorial Program Assistant: Courtney Allen

Technical Editor: George Nikias, MD

Editorial Manager: Jennifer Ehrlich

Editorial Assistant: Nadine Bell

Cover Photos:
©Ed Pritchard/Getty Images/Stone

Cartoons: Rich Tennant
(www.the5thwave.com)

Composition Services

Project Coordinator: Michael Kruzil

Layout and Graphics: Andrea Dahl, Lauren Goddard, Denny Hager, Stephanie D. Jumper, Barry Offringa, Jacque Roth, Heather Ryan

Special Art: Kathryn Born

Proofreaders: Jessica Kramer, Charles Spencer, TECHBOOKS Production Services

Indexer: TECHBOOKS Production Services

Publishing and Editorial for Consumer Dummies

    Diane Graves Steele, Vice President and Publisher, Consumer Dummies

    Joyce Pepple, Acquisitions Director, Consumer Dummies

    Kristin A. Cocks, Product Development Director, Consumer Dummies

    Michael Spring, Vice President and Publisher, Travel

    Brice Gosnell, Associate Publisher, Travel

    Kelly Regan, Editorial Director, Travel

Publishing for Technology Dummies

    Andy Cummings, Vice President and Publisher, Dummies Technology/General User

Composition Services

    Gerry Fahey, Vice President of Production Services

    Debbie Stailey, Director of Composition Services

Contents at a Glance

Table of Contents

Foreword

● ●

I'm thrilled to be writing the foreword for *Living with Hepatitis C For Dummies*. Nina L. Paul, PhD, has written a comprehensive guide to living with this illness. Nina has studied epidemiology, immunology, and viruses extensively, and her vast knowledge and experience have made her the ideal author for this book. She covers every issue of living with and managing hepatitis C — from diagnosis to treatment. The *For Dummies* series of books has been around for quite some time, and it's refreshing to see hepatitis C written about in such an insightful way. Having a well-written, user-friendly book that can educate people with this diagnosis is a godsend.

I know firsthand how important it is to have a guide like this. When you have hepatitis C, it seems all you have are questions and not many answers. Being diagnosed with this illness can create much confusion and fear, and you may feel powerless over the disease. By learning all you can about hepatitis C and how best to deal with it, your overwhelming anxiety is lessened. Reading *Living with Hepatitis C For Dummies* can do just that!

Many people have no symptoms from hepatitis C, yet they often worry about the uncertainty of what the disease will bring in the future. In addition, hepatitis C patients often deal with the stigma surrounding the disease. A large portion of our society knows nothing about hepatitis C, and those who do often have many misconceptions. This book not only educates the patient with clear, concise, and accurate information, but it can also be shared with family and friends to help them understand what the patient is dealing with. Having any chronic illness creates many challenges, but you can learn to face them head on and learn how to deal with them in a more positive way. When you arm yourself with knowledge, you empower yourself and ultimately gain some sense of control over your illness. You may not be able to control the outcome, but you have the power to control how you deal with it. The information and knowledge this book provides will help to give you the power to face this disease head on.

When I first started running support groups for hepatitis C patients, I saw a great number of people with many misconceptions about the disease. Much has been learned since the early '90s. Early on, I saw many people struggle through interferon monotherapy, yet I saw very few people respond to the treatment regimen. Over time, with the addition of ribavirin, I saw many more patients respond and remain virus free at the end of treatment. The next leap forward was pegylated interferon. As the research chronicled a much better response rate, I saw those results firsthand with the patients in my support groups. Witnessing this great advance in hepatitis C treatment has been wonderful, and I feel very fortunate to work with patients who are benefiting from these advances. But the most important message here is that there is hope for someday living a life free of the hepatitis C virus. Of course, not everyone can take treatment for various reasons, and not all of those who do will respond. With ongoing research, many more drug regimens will be used, and ultimately many, many more people will be cured.

My personal journey with this disease began in 1994 with acute hepatitis C. As an RN, I knew what hepatitis was, but beyond that, I knew very little. If this book were available at the time of my diagnosis, it would have been much easier to understand the disease and overcome the fear and uncertainty. Just like everyone else with this illness, I wish that I didn't have hepatitis C. However, the glass is still half full for me, and it can be for you, too. I have hepatitis C, but it's just one aspect of my life, of which there are many. It is possible to deal with adversity with grace and dignity, and out of this struggle comes personal growth. When you have hepatitis C, it changes some of the ways that you view your life and the decisions you must make, but you can learn to deal with the changes this disease brings about. Living with hepatitis C is an ongoing journey, and you will get all the information you need to move forward in this journey right here in this book. Bravo, Nina Paul, for writing *Living with Hepatitis C For Dummies!* It's the ultimate hepatitis C guide, and I applaud your efforts!

— Gina Pollichino, RN

Introduction

● ●

Millions of people in the United States and all over the world have been infected with hepatitis C. Many don't even know they have it, because symptoms may not appear for decades.

The sooner you know that you have hepatitis C, the sooner you can begin medical treatment and start making lifestyle changes to protect others from infection and keep yourself healthy.

Hepatitis C infects the liver and causes a range of disease from none-at-all to life-threatening liver disease that can only be treated with a liver transplant. Most people fall within these two extremes.

Hepatitis C virus spreads through contact with infected blood. You could've received hepatitis C from a blood transfusion or from sharing any type of needle or sharp instrument for medical, cosmetic, or drug use.

But how you got your hepatitis C is nowhere near as important as what you're doing now to help yourself stay well. Use this book to help you build a support network and make *informed* choices about your healthcare and lifestyle.

About This Book

While writing this book, I've tried to focus on the friendly advice given to me by a woman with hepatitis C:

> *"I want choices. I need info. I want to defuse my fears. And please, keep it simple."*

I've also hung my hat on the fact that every individual facing hepatitis C is just that — *an individual.* You may be young or old, male or female. You're of a different race, ethnic group, or nationality than others. You have different responses to different medications, as well as different personal preferences on the types of medications you'll take. You have different levels of healthcare due to different finances and locations. In this book, I present various options and choices so that you can find the ones that work best for you.

Throughout this book, I emphasize the value of a positive attitude, because it helps you deal with the healthcare system, reduces stress, and just plain makes you feel better (as well as everyone around you).

I believe that it's important to dispel myths about hepatitis C and eliminate prejudices and stigmas against people with the virus. The best offense against closed-mindedness is information. So I help clear up any misconceptions and questions you may have about the disease, and I give you information, tips, and resources for dealing with negativity that you may face because of your illness.

Conventions Used in This Book

Throughout the book, I use certain words interchangeably:

- ✔ In some places, the doctor is a *he,* and in other places, a *she.*
- ✔ When I write *healthcare providers* or *healthcare practitioners,* I usually mean your doctor (physician). But this term includes professional nurse practitioners, physician assistants, nutritionists, and naturopaths.
- ✔ Hepatitis C is also called hep C, hep C virus, and sometimes HCV (hepatitis C virus)
- ✔ When I refer to medications, I usually present the generic name first, followed by the brand name in parentheses.

To help you navigate through this book, I use the following typographical conventions:

- ✔ *Italic* is used for emphasis and to highlight new words or terms that are defined in the text.
- ✔ **Boldfaced** text is used to indicate keywords in bulleted lists or the action parts of numbered steps.
- ✔ Monofont is used for Web addresses.
- ✔ Sidebars are shaded gray boxes that contain text that's interesting to know but not necessarily critical to your understanding of the chapter or section topic.

Finally, I aim to provide the most accurate statistics on hepatitis C. But numbers change, depending on a large number of factors, such as the specific medications, the different types of people a study looked at, and so on. So consider the numbers I give you as approximations.

What You're Not to Read

Each of you has different needs and interests, so read the chapters that apply to you. If you don't know a child with hepatitis C, for example, skip the chapter on children. The same thing applies to sidebars that are asides to the main topic and information marked with the Technical Stuff icon. On the other hand, you're free to read all of the text, if you want. I happen to think it's all great information (but I could be a little biased on that matter).

Foolish Assumptions

All writers have to make assumptions about their audience, and I'm no different. While writing this book, I've assumed the following:

- ✔ You're not really a dummy, or else you wouldn't have picked up this book.
- ✔ You have come to this book to find reliable, up-to-date information on hepatitis C in a clear and readable format.
- ✔ You want some background on the virus and your liver so you can get a handle on what's going on in your body.
- ✔ You want to learn about alternative treatments, whether you actually use them or not.
- ✔ You want to know the pros and cons of interferon treatment.
- ✔ You will at least think about dropping some of those bad habits, if doing so will help you stay healthy.

How This Book Is Organized

To help you navigate through the different aspects of hepatitis C, I've separated the information into parts: basic background information; medical information; lifestyle and living issues; and specific chapters for children, women, minorities, and family and friends.

Part 1: Understanding and Exposing Hepatitis C

You may be wondering what the heck is going on inside your body when you have hepatitis C. In this part, I present the basic science about hepatitis C. You can read about the hepatitis C virus and other hepatitis viruses, how these viruses are transmitted, and how to protect others. I also explain how hepatitis C infects and harms your hard-working liver, and describe the symptoms and how the disease progresses.

Part II: Diagnosing and Treating the Disease

In this part, I explain the different types of doctors who can treat hepatitis C and offer advice on how you can find and work with a doctor. I discuss the different laboratory tests that you undergo before a diagnosis is made, and give you information on conventional and alternative hepatitis C therapies, which you can use to help you decide on treatment. This part is where you also can find a discussion of liver transplants.

Part III: Living a Good Life with Hep C

This part offers advice on choosing healthy foods, exercising regularly, reducing stress, and avoiding substances and lifestyle choices that will further harm your liver. I also explain how to get the support you need, discuss your hep C with others, manage your work life, and handle financial issues related to dealing with this chronic illness.

Part IV: Considering Different Groups with Hepatitis C

Anyone can get hepatitis C, and in this part, I look at specific issues related to children, women, men, different ethnic groups, and other special groups with hepatitis C. Another important group is the family and friends of people with hepatitis C, and I devote a whole chapter to helping these folks.

Part V: The Part of Tens

In this classic part of the *For Dummies* books, you can find tips about traveling when you have hepatitis C and getting a good night's sleep. I also list resources that you can turn to for more information about hepatitis C.

Icons Used in This Book

Throughout the book, you'll see small illustrations to the left of some text. These are called icons, and they alert you to the type of information presented.

This fine piece of art alerts you to practical information and insight that you can put to use.

The Remember icon marks information that's so important, you don't ever want to forget it.

When I discuss something that could be dangerous to your health, I use the Warning icon.

This icon indicates you're entering a jargon zone that you may wish to skip or where you may want to tread carefully. It's great information, don't get me wrong, but not reading it won't affect your grasp on the matter at hand.

When you see this icon, you need to consult your physician about a particular matter.

I use this icon to let you know when you should obtain and file away copies of important medical information.

Where to Go from Here

You're ready to delve into the meat of the book now. Like all *For Dummies* books, this book is designed to let you get in and get out — you can start reading anywhere. Each chapter is a self-contained bundle of information, so using the table of contents, you can head straight to the chapter that best meets your needs. Or you can start with Chapter 1 and read straight through.

Here are my suggestions to enhance your use of this book:

- ✔ Have your test results and other medical information handy as you go through the book.
- ✔ Start a healthcare notebook or binder of the information.
- ✔ Write down any questions that come up to ask your doctor, support group, or spouse.

Remember, many other people with hepatitis C are walking the same steps, and you can find them, if you like, in support groups (see Chapter 14). Good luck in your journey to live well with hepatitis C!

Part I
Understanding and Exposing Hepatitis C

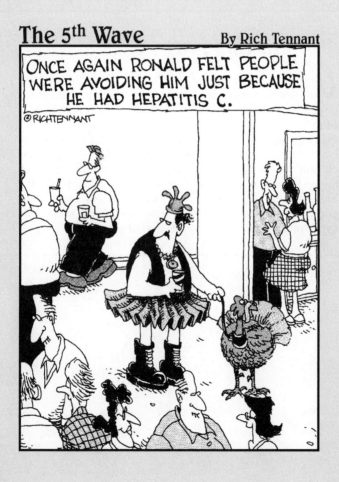

The 5th Wave   By Rich Tennant

ONCE AGAIN RONALD FELT PEOPLE WE·RE AVOIDING HIM JUST BECAUSE HE HAD HEPATITIS C.

In this part . . .

When you have hep C, you're not alone. Millions of people around the world have been exposed to infected blood, causing an epidemic of hepatitis C. Like other hepatitis viruses, hepatitis C infects the liver. In many people, hepatitis C has the unfortunate feature of staying in the body for decades and becoming a long-term chronic illness. Hep C has a long list of symptoms, depending on the damage to your liver. In this part, I describe the basic biology of the hepatitis C virus, your immune system, and the workings of your wonderful liver. I also explain the symptoms and disease progression of hepatitis C.

Chapter 1

Conquering Hepatitis C

● ●

In This Chapter

▶ Looking at the complications and symptoms of the disease

▶ Finding out how hep C is transmitted

▶ Testing, testing, testing

▶ Taking care of yourself

▶ Managing your finances and your medical records

▶ Making the best decisions for you

● ●

Hepatitis C is called an epidemic because of the numbers of people infected. In the United States, almost 4 million people have hepatitis C virus. In Canada, the number is 240,000. In the entire world, at least 170 million people are currently infected. Hepatitis C virus has infected so many people because of the way that it spreads — through contact with infected blood.

If you or a loved one has been recently diagnosed with hepatitis C, and if you're like most folks, you probably have a lot of questions and a fair number of fears. This book can help answer those questions and, in the process, quiet the fears.

Hepatitis C does *not* have to be a death sentence. Getting medical treatment; staying away from alcohol and other dangers to your liver; and otherwise taking good care of your body, mind, and spirit can allow you to live long and live well.

In this chapter, I introduce the essential concepts about living with the hepatitis C virus. My goal is to quickly answer the most pressing questions you may have and let you know where you can find more information on each matter in the rest of the book.

How Hepatitis C Is Spread

Hepatitis C is a virus, and it spreads from person to person through infected blood. Everyone should know how hepatitis C virus is transmitted so they can take measures to protect themselves.

In the United States and other developed countries, the blood supply wasn't tested until 1992, so if you got a blood transfusion or underwent any type of organ transplant before then, you could've gotten the hep C virus.

The blood supplies in developed Western countries are now safe, but this isn't the case around the world. In developing or transitional countries (as defined by the World Health Organization, or WHO), reuse of injection equipment for medical procedures is the major source of new infections.

Here are the main ways that hepatitis C can now spread in the United States and other developed countries:

- ✔ Use of shared equipment for drug use, tattoos, or piercing.
- ✔ Mother-to-child transmission.
- ✔ Sexual transmission.
- ✔ Sharing items such as toothbrushes or razors with someone with hepatitis C.
- ✔ Occupational exposure.

To read more about transmission of this virus and how to protect others, check out Chapter 2. If you feel that you have a risk factor for hepatitis C virus, go see your doctor, and get a hepatitis C test (I discuss the tests in Chapter 6).

Hepatitis C timeline in United States

Hepatitis C was initially called hepatitis non-A non-B before it was identified. Here's a list of some milestones in the identification of hep C, protection of the United States blood supply, and treatment of hepatitis C.

1980s 242,000 new infections of hepatitis C occurred per year.

1987 Clotting factor protected (because of precautions against HIV).

1989 Hepatitis C virus was identified.

1992 Blood supply in the United States first tested for hepatitis C.

1996 Interferon first used in treatment of hepatitis C.

1998 Interferon plus ribavirin became standard treatment.

2001 25,000 new infections of hepatitis C.

2002 Pegylated interferon plus ribavirin became standard treatment.

Getting Tested for Hepatitis C

Hepatitis C is a silent virus; most people don't know they have the virus until decades after infection. You can find out if you've been exposed to hepatitis C by taking a blood test.

In addition to the risk factors I outline in the previous section, you should get tested for hepatitis C if you've ever been on long-term kidney dialysis or have signs of liver disease.

In Chapter 6, I cover all the tests and the possible results in detail. But basically, hep C tests come in two forms, both of which involve drawing some blood:

- **Antibody test:** The first level of tests looks for the immune response to the virus, called *antibody*. The antibody test tells if you've ever seen the virus, even in the past. It doesn't tell you if have the virus now.

- **RNA tests:** More-direct tests of the virus look for the virus component called RNA, or ribonucleic acid. The RNA test tells if you have the virus right now and how much you have (viral load or quantitative test).

After you know you have hepatitis C, see a liver specialist to get an expert evaluation of your condition. Turn to Chapter 5 for tips on choosing and communicating with your doctor.

Describing the Disease

Hepatitis means inflammation (*itis*) of the liver (*hepa*). The subject of this book is hepatitis C, but actually, a number of viruses infect the liver and cause liver disease — and they're all called *hepatitis viruses*. You can read more about the differences between these viruses in Chapter 2, but for the moment, I concentrate on the one that brought you here.

Hepatitis C around the world

Hepatitis C affects millions of people around the globe — rich and poor. Calling hepatitis C a "viral time bomb," the World Health Organization (WHO) estimates that

✔ About 3 percent of the world's population is infected with hep C.

✔ 3 to 4 million new infections occur each year.

✔ Around 170 million people are chronically infected and risk getting cirrhosis and/or liver cancer.

Chronic infections can be treated with medication in developed countries (see the "Choosing treatments" section in this chapter), but unfortunately, the cost of such medications is too high for most of the millions of people living in countries with fewer financial resources.

The numbers

Everyone responds differently to hepatitis C virus. If you've been infected with hepatitis C virus, you want to know what'll happen to you. Your doctor is the best person to advise you on your particular situation. But I'll present some numbers, here and throughout the book. *Remember:* These numbers are only estimates.

Of the people exposed to hepatitis C virus,

✔ 15 to 25 percent clear (get rid of) the virus when they first get infected.

✔ 75 to 85 percent develop a long-term, or *chronic,* infection.

About 20 percent of the people who have a long-term chronic infection get *cirrhosis.* Cirrhosis can occur 10 or 20 years or more after you're first infected. After you have cirrhosis, you're at risk of getting the most serious illness — liver failure or liver cancer.

If you develop liver failure or have liver cancer, the best treatment is a liver transplant (see Chapter 9). Between 1 to 5 percent of people with hepatitis C virus will die from the disease.

The liver

The hepatitis C virus infects liver cells. For most people with hepatitis C, the main problem is how hepatitis C hurts your liver. The liver processes practically every single thing you eat, drink, or otherwise absorb into your body. It makes proteins, filters out waste and toxins, stores sugars and vitamins, and converts foods and drugs into usable substances. (See Chapter 4 for more information on the liver and its normal functions.)

The disease

To see the extent of liver disease, your doctor will perform blood tests. You may already have had an ALT (alanine transferase) test, which is commonly used to look for liver damage but is by no means the only test. (See Chapter 7 for a description of other tests that look for liver damage or changes in liver function.)

You doctor will probably suggest a liver biopsy, which gives a direct picture of your liver. The liver biopsy can show two types of damage to your liver from hepatitis C:

- ✔ **Inflammation:** This earlier stage of damage is reversible.

- ✔ **Scarring (fibrosis):** Most experts agree that scarring is probably somewhat reversible in early stages, but continued scarring damages the liver and isn't reversible.

Inflammation causes the disease called *hepatitis,* which gives you symptoms of hepatitis C, but your disease isn't life-threatening unless you get *cirrhosis.* Scarring prevents your liver from performing its crucial jobs to keep your body functioning. When scarring covers most of the liver, you get *cirrhosis.* There are two types of cirrhosis:

- ✔ **Compensated cirrhosis:** Even though you have cirrhosis, your liver is still performing its tasks.

- ✔ **Decompensated cirrhosis:** This is another name for *end-stage liver disease* or *liver failure.* Here, your liver is no longer working properly. You'll die from the damage to your liver, unless you get a liver transplant.

Liver cancer (hepatocellular carcinoma) is a life-threatening disease that sometimes occurs in people with cirrhosis. Your doctor will give you an ultrasound or other imaging test to see if there is evidence of liver tumors (see Chapter 7).

If you have liver cancer (only for some stages, though) or end-stage liver disease, a liver transplant can save your life. Read about treatments for liver disease in Chapter 8 and about liver transplants in Chapter 9.

The symptoms

If you have chronic hepatitis C, your symptoms can be bothersome and, in some cases, debilitating. Chronic hepatitis C disease has many symptoms. The most common are fatigue (which is more than tiredness and persists even after a good night's sleep), nausea and vomiting, muscle and joint aches, itchy skin, fluid retention, brain fog (loss of concentration, ability to focus, or remember), and depression. In Chapter 4, I provide a longer list of symptoms and outline the progression of hepatitis C disease.

Along with problems with your liver, you may have other illnesses that are associated with hepatitis C. These are called *extrahepatic diseases* because they're not strictly liver (hepatic) diseases and include diseases of the skin or kidneys. In Chapter 4, I describe a few of the other types of illnesses you may experience with hepatitis C.

Fighting Hepatitis C

Wherever you are in the battle to heal from hepatitis C, you hold the keys to preventing further liver damage.

Seek the advice and care of qualified healthcare practitioners. I give some tips on finding practitioners in Chapter 5 and on evaluating healthcare choices in Chapter 10.

Choosing treatments

The medical fight against hepatitis C is evolving. At this time, the primary recommended treatment by the U.S. Food and Drug Administration (FDA) for chronic hepatitis C is a combination of two drugs — *interferon* and *ribavirin*. These drugs can stop the hep C virus from growing in your body. The form of interferon that's currently used is called *pegylated interferon,* or the shortened version, *peginterferon.* Therefore, you'll see the treatment referred to as *peginterferon plus ribavirin therapy.* Got all that? Just think: There are more rather strange names waiting for you in Chapter 8, where I discuss this and other Western medical treatments.

But not everyone with hepatitis C undergoes drug treatment. The decision whether to pursue this path now, later, or never is one that you'll make with the help of your doctor. Among other things to consider about combination treatment (see Chapter 8) are the following:

✔ Combination interferon treatment can be long and costly, and has the possibility of severe side effects.

✔ Between 50 and 80 percent of people who go through treatment have success in that the hepatitis C virus becomes undetectable in their body for at least six months after treatment. Some doctors call this a "cure" because it can halt further damage from hepatitis C virus.

Alternative medical systems such as Eastern or traditional Chinese medicine, ayurvedic medicine, and homeopathic and naturopathic medicine also offer treatments that can be used instead of or alongside Western medicine and that are less likely to result in severe side effects. These alternatives, however, are also less likely (as determined by the FDA) to eliminate the virus (see Chapter 10).

Medical care is increasingly incorporating both Western (traditional) medicine and Eastern (alternative or complementary) medicine in what's called an integrated approach to healthcare.

Choosing healthy living

Regardless of whether you can take medical treatment or whether it's successful in eliminating your virus, you can still fight the effects of hep C by making wise lifestyle choices, including the following suggestions:

✔ **Eat healthful foods.** Your liver and immune system need nutrients from food to fight the virus and build new liver cells (read about healthy eating in Chapter 11). Avoiding fatty, junk-type foods will reduce symptoms of hep C.

✔ **Avoid toxins.** Products such as paint thinners, chemical cleaners, pesticides, and many household cleaning products are especially harmful for people with hep C. (See Chapter 12 for more on different types of toxins to stay away from.)

✔ **Give up dangerous addictive habits.** Say no to alcohol, smoking, and illegal drugs. Alcohol is especially damaging to your liver. If you need help (and most people do) to end these habits, check with your doctor or look into a substance-abuse program (see Chapter 12 for the details).

✔ **Take all medications with care.** Some medicines, including prescriptions and the over-the-counter variety, can harm your liver (see Chapter 12). Check with your healthcare practitioner to make sure they're not hurting your liver.

What you put into your body is one aspect of staying healthy. Also important is what you do with your body. Movement of some sort, whether it's strenuous exercise, gentle stretching, or a mind-body-spirit movement such as T'ai Chi or Yoga, is essential for good health. Exercising your body keeps you limber and helps fight depression and fatigue, two common symptoms of hepatitis C. Chapter 13 focuses on the power of movement to help you feel better and reduce stress.

Letting others help you

Living with a chronic illness can feel frustrating, scary, and lonely. You don't have to live on an emotional roller coaster. Build a support team that includes the following members:

- ✔ **Your physicians:** See Chapter 5 for tips on finding and communicating with a liver specialist and other doctors.

- ✔ **Friends, family, and neighbors:** All these folks can help out when you're not feeling well. Chapter 19 talks about how friends and family can help you.

- ✔ **Spouse or partner:** Discuss your concerns with your loved ones. See Chapter 15 for tips on communicating with your partner and strengthening other important relationships.

- ✔ **Mental health professional:** When the going gets too tough to handle on your own, seek professional help. I give some tips for finding a therapist in Chapter 14.

- ✔ **A support group:** You can get information and comfort from discussions with other people with hepatitis C — either in person or on the Internet. Chapter 14 tells you how to find a support group near you.

Depression is a serious side effect of hepatitis C virus and the medical treatment (interferon). Don't neglect the signs of depression (see Chapter 14). A professional can determine if you would benefit from an antidepressant and/or counseling.

Getting Financial Support

Chronic hepatitis C symptoms can make you unable to work at your usual pace or job, or even cause you to become disabled. To get the most benefit from your health insurance, read your policy carefully, and ask questions. You don't necessarily have to tell your boss you have hepatitis C. But if you want to be protected against discrimination, your employer must know about your hepatitis C. Sounds like a Catch-22, doesn't it? See Chapter 16 for more information on facing the financial challenges of hep C and the challenges you may find in the workplace.

You need to know more about your insurance than the name and phone number of the company. You need to know the nitty-gritty details:

✔ What's covered and what's not, including medications, tests, hospital visits, and mental health care

✔ The type of co-payments or deductibles you have

✔ The doctors you can visit

✔ How to change doctors

✔ A yearly maximum amount that's covered

✔ Coverage of liver transplants

If you don't have health insurance, you can get help with medical treatment through clinics or Medicaid or by contacting the pharmaceutical companies that make peginterferon plus ribavirin (see Chapter 22).

Staying Organized with a Hep C Notebook

Keep your medical information and health records in a safe place. You may need to show this documentation if you visit new health-care practitioners or if you apply for life insurance or Social Security disability. I provide a complete description of how to build a hep C notebook in Chapter 5, but for now, here are the types of information to save or record:

✔ Copies of all tests, which you should request at the time of the test or from your doctor who ordered the test

✔ Dates and outcomes of all doctor visits

✔ A running list of your symptoms

✔ Medications, dates taken, side effects, and results

✔ Vitamins, herbs, and over-the-counter medicines you take (see Chapter 12)

You, and trusted friends or family members, are the true gatekeepers of your health plan. I'm not talking about a health insurance plan, but a plan to get better. Use this book to help you make the choices that are right for you.

You're More Than a Statistic

I kept the idea of individuality in mind as I wrote this book, and I want you to keep it in mind, too. Every person with hepatitis C is a unique individual. From your biological makeup to your lifestyle, you're different from the next person.

Hep C isn't a one-size-fits-all disease. There are real differences in the way different people's disease shows up or the way they respond to treatment. So I provide specific information for children, women and men, African Americans and Latinos, and other folks in Part IV of this book. Make sure that your doctor has experience not only in treating people with hepatitis C, but also in treating people who are similar to you in age, ethnicity, lifestyle, and so on.

Even though I give you facts, figures, and information from studies that are performed on *groups* of people, I still want you to remember that you are more than a number.

Therefore, because you're you, your doctor and other healthcare professionals who have an intimate knowledge of your specific situation are your best source of information. This book is meant to provide you with the information that will let you carry on informed conversations with your healthcare professionals and family members and be your own best advocate.

Chapter 2

Talking about Transmission

Simply put, any type of activity that allows the exchange of blood between people can serve as a way to spread hepatitis C. Although the injection of illegal drugs is a primary means of transmission, it's not the only way to get the hepatitis C virus. Likewise, to *avoid giving* hepatitis C virus to others means keeping your blood safely away from other people. In this chapter, I discuss how transmission of the hepatitis C virus through blood occurs so you can try to understand how you got the virus and make sure that you don't spread it to anyone else.

But the hepatitis C virus isn't the only virus that can cause hepatitis. There are different hepatitis viruses (from A to E), each of which has a different type of transmission. If you're infected with more than one hepatitis virus, the result can be more-serious symptoms and different treatment approaches. In this chapter, I also outline each of these viruses so that you know where hepatitis C fits into the scheme of things and you can learn how to protect yourself. *Hint:* See your doctor about getting vaccinated against hepatitis A and B.

Tracing Hepatitis C Transmission

You'll have many questions when you find out you have hepatitis C. One of the most common is "How did I get this virus?" You may not find out about your hep C infection until months or decades after you were infected, and when all is said and done, about 10 percent of folks aren't sure how they got infected.

You may be upset or angry about how you got hep C. You're not alone. Get support to talk about your feelings (see Chapter 14). But to heal from hep C, how you got the virus isn't as important as what you do to treat yourself *now,* which I cover in Parts II and III.

Hepatitis C is transmitted by close contact with blood that's contaminated with the hep C virus. The following sections outline the various ways you might have gotten hep C.

Blood transfusions and other medical procedures

Because hepatitis C is spread through infected blood, any medical procedure in which you received a blood transfusion or blood product, or were exposed to even the slightest trace of blood, could have put you at risk of infection.

Tests for the antibody (see Chapter 6) to the hepatitis C virus became available in the early 1990s, and blood in the United States and Canada was tested from that time onward. July 1992 is the official date in the USA from which all blood sources were tested for hepatitis C. The U.S. Centers for Disease Control and Prevention (CDC) reports that the likelihood of getting hep C from the blood supply now is less than 1 chance per 1,000,000 blood units donated.

Here are other medical procedures or products that may have put you at risk:

- **Long-term kidney dialysis:** Dialysis is considered a risk factor because of the possibility of blood being present on the dialysis machine.

- **Reused needle for vaccination, acupuncture, or other medical procedure:** The needle could have traces of contaminated blood.

- **Organ transplant:** The organ may have been contaminated with hepatitis C virus from the donor. Donors are now tested for hepatitis C virus.

- **Receiving blood-clotting factor for hemophilia before 1987:** Starting in 1987, the factors were treated against HIV, which also protected against hepatitis C virus.

Blood supplies in the United States, Canada, and other developed countries are now tested against hepatitis C, but this isn't necessarily the case in developing parts of the world. Keep this fact in mind if you travel to or live in certain countries (see Chapter 20 for travel tips).

Injected street drugs

In the United States and other developed countries, injecting illegal drugs is the leading source of current hep C infection. If you've ever shared a needle or any part of the drug works, which includes cotton, water, spoons, and anything else that may contain blood from someone else — *even if you didn't see any blood* — you may have been exposed to hepatitis C.

Just using illegal drugs with shared syringes or works one time is enough to get the hep C virus.

Healthcare professionals who treat people with hep C shouldn't judge you for your past or current behavior that may have caused your hep C. Read Chapter 5 for advice on finding a doctor whom you can work with. If you're still using drugs, see Chapter 12 for advice on how to deal with your addiction.

Intranasal drug use

If you ever used straws or paper money to snort cocaine or other drugs into your nose, you may have been exposed to hep C virus. Blood can be exchanged in this way if the nasal membranes bleed onto the shared item.

Mother to child

A woman who has hepatitis C virus in her blood has a low but definite risk of passing the virus to her child. On average, 5 percent of children born to mothers with hepatitis C virus become infected with the virus. There are no reports of transmission from mother to child through breastfeeding. However, if a woman's nipples are cracked or bleeding, avoiding breastfeeding is the best course of action. See Chapter 17 for information about hepatitis C infection in children.

Sexual activity

Studies have shown that sexual transmission of hep C is rare but possible. This topic has elicited some controversy, because some studies show virtually no transmission of hep C virus between men and women in long-term monogamous relationships. But it's believed that the risk of sexual transmission increases

✔ If you have multiple sex partners.

✔ If you have sexually transmitted diseases.

✔ If you're exposed to blood during sex.

For tips on preventing sexual transmission, see the "Protecting others from getting infected" section later in the chapter and check out Chapter 15 for information on dealing with many aspects of relationships, including sexual activity.

Sharing personal items

Things like toothbrushes, razors, cuticle scissors, and other personal items that come into contact with infected blood could transmit hep C from one person to another.

Tattoos and piercings

Reusing needles or other sharp tools for tattoos or body piercings could spread hep C infection. It's also believed that using the same tattoo inkpot, even with fresh needles, could spread hep C. For the most part, scientific studies haven't found tattoos or piercings to be a major cause of hepatitis C infection in the United States. But the risk can't be ruled out as a potential source of infection, especially if you had a tattoo or piercing in an unsanitary setting, such as in the military or in prison.

Occupational exposure

You risk exposure to hepatitis C if your work puts you in contact with potentially infected blood. Healthcare workers (phlebotomists, nurses, doctors, dentists, emergency medical technicians, and others), public safety workers (fire-service and law enforcement), and corrections officers may be exposed to blood on the job. Accidental needlestick injury is the most likely cause of exposure to hepatitis C.

If you've been recently exposed to hepatitis C virus, seek medical attention (see Chapter 5) immediately, because early treatment is effective in eradicating the virus (see Chapter 8).

Ways that hep C is not transmitted

Hepatitis C virus is *not* transmitted during everyday activities and casual contact. Hepatitis is transmitted through exposure to *blood*. The hepatitis C virus is *not* spread in the following ways:

- ✔ Sneezing or coughing
- ✔ Hugging or kissing
- ✔ Sharing forks or other eating utensils
- ✔ Sharing drinking glasses
- ✔ Through food or water
- ✔ Holding hands
- ✔ Breastfeeding

Protecting Others from Getting Infected

However you got your hep C, be responsible, and take precautions to prevent others from getting infected. The goal here is to achieve a balance between being aware that you have an infectious virus but not becoming paranoid. Hepatitis C is transmitted through blood. Unless you're a vampire who regularly deals with blood, I assume that your blood is normally well inside your body. To be absolutely careful and guard against infecting others, follow these tips:

- ✔ Don't donate blood. But you may be able to donate body organs to other hep C-infected people.

- ✔ Don't let anyone else use your razor, toothbrush, manicure scissors, or other personal-care items that may have blood on them. Be especially careful about keeping these items away from children. Keep your toothbrush and toothpaste, which may have some blood on it from your toothbrush, in a separate drawer or cabinet.

- ✔ Cover open cuts or sores on your skin with bandages until they have healed. Carry bandages on you, in your purse, or in your vehicle so that you're always prepared.

- ✔ Carefully dispose of anything that has been exposed to your blood (from menstruation or a wound, for example).

- ✔ If you use illegal drugs, don't share your needles or any paraphernalia with anyone else. This precaution will also protect you from getting other viruses, such as hepatitis B or HIV.

In addition, be responsible in your sexual activity.

If you're in a monogamous relationship, your partner may want to get tested. Sexual transmission in these situations has been found to be rare. But you may want to start using a latex condom.

Discuss sexual transmission with your healthcare practitioner and your partner (see Chapter 15).

Your risk of spreading hepatitis C is greater if you have multiple partners or are exposed to blood during sex. You may be exposed to blood during sexual activity in these situations:

- ✔ When a woman is menstruating
- ✔ During rough sex in which one person bleeds
- ✔ During anal sex, which may damage the lining of the rectum
- ✔ When you or your partner has an open sore on the genitals (from herpes or another sexually transmitted disease)

Hep C isn't known to be spread through oral sex, but it's theoretically possible if contact with blood occurs, which could happen if you have sores on your genitals, bleeding gums, or abrasions from shaving. To prevent this, try to avoid shaving, flossing, or brushing your teeth before having sex. (Try a breath mint or gargling to freshen your breath.)

Use male or female condoms to reduce your chances of getting sexually transmitted diseases like HIV, gonorrhea, or syphilis, as well as to protect from spreading hep C virus. There's also a product called a *dental dam* (a latex sheet) that can be used during oral sex. Latex condoms are best studied for their ability to prevent spread of virus, but some people have allergies to latex, in which case polyurethane is the next-best option.

Safer sex means getting information on how sex can spread disease or cause pregnancy, being honest with yourself and your partner about your sexual desires and your risks for infection, and making decisions for protection that work for both you and your partner.

Decisions about sex are individual, and your healthcare provider can help you understand your situation (the infectious diseases you have and how your particular sexual activities put you at risk) so you can best protect yourself and your partner.

Reviewing the Hepatitis Virus ABCs

As I discuss in Chapter 1, the term *hepatitis* simply means inflammation of the liver. But when you're talking about hepatitis C, you're talking about *viral hepatitis,* and hep C isn't the only form of hepatitis caused by a virus. (Check out the "Examining other causes of hepatitis" sidebar in this chapter for information on nonviral forms of hepatitis.)

So far, five different viruses have been found that cause hepatitis, and they're named with letters: Hepatitis A virus causes hepatitis A; hepatitis B virus causes hepatitis B; hepatitis C virus causes hepatitis C; and hepatitis E virus causes hepatitis E. Hepatitis D virus is a special case, because it can't infect you unless you also have hepatitis B virus. The following sections provide a bit more detail about each virus.

The different types of viral hepatitis have similar features but also important differences. Depending on the hepatitis virus, the disease may be temporary — an *acute* form, which lasts less than a year. With hepatitis B or C, though, infection can become *chronic* and last for decades, or life, unless you undergo successful treatment against the virus.

Examining other causes of hepatitis

Agents other than viruses can cause Inflammation of the liver, which is what the word *hepatitis* means. Viral hepatitis is more common than most of these other types of hepatitis, but I simply include this list so you know what else can cause hepatitis besides viruses.

✔ *Alcoholic hepatitis* is caused by alcohol damage to the liver. Alcohol damage starts as alcoholic fatty liver disease, which can turn into hepatitis. If you continue to consume alcohol, you can get cirrhosis of the liver.

✔ *Autoimmune hepatitis* is a disease in which the body's immune system attacks liver cells. This disease may be inherited through your genes, and it affects women more than men.

✔ *Drug-induced hepatitis* is caused by a severe liver reaction to over-the-counter or prescription drugs. Some medicines can cause serious complications in the liver when taken improperly, or even in some cases when taken properly. I list some of these drugs in Chapter 12.

✔ *Toxic hepatitis* is caused by toxic chemical damage to the liver. This can happen from an accidental exposure on the job or in the home to chemicals such as cleaning fluids or pesticides. Poisonous mushrooms, when eaten in error, can also cause toxic hepatitis.

People with hep C should avoid alcohol, dangerous drugs, and chemicals to prevent further damaging the liver. See Chapter 12 for more information on avoiding dangerous substances.

You're considered to be *infectious* if you have the virus and can possibly pass it to others — even if you don't have any symptoms. To read about hepatitis C symptoms, some of which are common to all viral hepatitis, see Chapter 4.

Hepatitis A virus

Hepatitis A (also called *infectious hepatitis*) was identified in 1973. Hepatitis A spreads through food or water that has been contaminated with infected feces (see Chapter 3 for more on how viruses are transmitted). You can get hepatitis A from:

- ✔ **Not washing your hands after exposure to feces:** Examples include not washing your hands after using the bathroom or changing a diaper.

- ✔ **Eating contaminated food:** This situation can occur with uncooked food and food prepared by someone who didn't wash his hands after using the toilet.

- ✔ **Drinking contaminated water:** Dealing with contaminated water could be a problem when traveling; see Chapter 20 for tips to avoid infection.

- ✔ **Sexual contact with someone who's infected:** Practice safer sex (see Chapter 15) and especially take care if you have anal or oral–anal sex.

Hepatitis A causes an acute infection. In the United States, 200,000 cases of hepatitis A are reported yearly, and a third of all people have already been exposed to hepatitis A virus at some point in their lives but may not have known it. If you've been exposed to hepatitis A in the past or gotten a vaccine, you'll be *immune,* or protected from future hepatitis A infection.

Hepatitis B virus

The hepatitis B virus (*serum hepatitis*) was found in 1963 and spreads through contact with infected body fluids (including saliva, vaginal fluid, and semen) and blood. You can get hepatitis B from

- ✔ Injection drug use

- ✔ Unprotected sex

- ✔ Transmission from mother to child during birth

- ✔ The razor or toothbrush of an infected person

- ✔ Occupational exposure of healthcare workers or emergency personnel to infected blood or body fluids

Hepatitis B can cause an acute or chronic infection, but chronic infection occurs in only approximately 5 percent of cases. A hepatitis B vaccine protects against hepatitis B (and hepatitis D; see the corresponding section below for more information on this virus that can make hepatitis B disease worse).

Hepatitis C virus

The hepatitis C virus was discovered in 1989. For decades before that, it was called "non-A non-B" hepatitis because researchers knew that it wasn't caused by the other known hepatitis viruses at the time. Hep C is transmitted through blood (see the section "Tracing Hepatitis C Transmission," earlier in this chapter), and 75 to 85 percent of people infected will have a chronic infection, which puts them at risk for cirrhosis, liver cancer, and liver failure over many decades of infection. No vaccine is available for hepatitis C, so prevention is the key to avoiding infection.

Hep C infection can last a lifetime, so you need to take good care of yourself physically, emotionally, and financially, as I explain in Part III of the book. Medical research is ongoing to develop more effective drugs with fewer side effects. Currently, combination therapy with two drugs — pegylated interferon and ribavirin — is the best treatment, but it doesn't work for everyone (see Chapter 8). Check out Chapter 3 for an in-depth discussion of the virus.

Hepatitis D virus

Hepatitis D was discovered in 1977 and is an incomplete virus that can't infect you on its own; it has to tag along with hepatitis B virus. When it does, it can produce more-severe hepatitis B disease. Transmission of hepatitis D is the same as for hepatitis B. Vaccination against hepatitis B prevents hepatitis D infection, too.

Hepatitis E virus

The hepatitis E virus was discovered in 1983 as another hepatitis virus that's transmitted through contamination of water with feces. Outbreaks of hepatitis E occur primarily in developing countries in Africa, Asia, and Central America due to unsanitary water supplies. Hepatitis E is rare in Canada, the United States, and other developed countries.

Hepatitis E is an acute infection. For some as-yet-unexplained reason, pregnant women appear to be at risk of a more severe disease when infected with hepatitis E. Follow the guidelines in Chapter 20 to avoid getting hepatitis E during foreign travel.

Other hepatitis viruses

Researchers believe that most people with viral hepatitis have one of the hepatitis viruses from A to E. But scientists are always on the lookout for new viruses that can cause disease. The viruses called hepatitis G virus (HGV), TTV (transfusion transmitted virus), and sentinel viruses (SEN) have all been discovered in the blood of people with hepatitis. But it's not absolutely clear that these viruses actually *cause* hepatitis. Hepatitis F is a name for a virus that's no longer thought to cause hepatitis.

Hepatitis virus co-infections

Having another hepatitis virus infection in addition to hepatitis C can cause more serious symptoms or difficulties in treatment:

- **Hepatitis A:** If you have hepatitis C and then get hepatitis A, you're more at risk of getting a severe and life-threatening form of hepatitis A called *fulminant hepatitis.* In other words, already having hepatitis C can make your hepatitis A disease worse. Get vaccinated against hepatitis A to avoid this problem.

- **Hepatitis B:** Hepatitis C and hepatitis B are both transmitted by blood, and both can cause a chronic long-term illness, although hep C is more likely than hep B to be chronic. Scientists are still trying to figure out how having both of these hepatitis viruses over a long period of time will affect your health. It's especially important that you see a liver-specialist doctor to help sort through the complexities of both of these hepatitis infections (for tips on finding a doctor, see Chapter 5). If you have hep C but don't currently have hepatitis B, get vaccinated against hepatitis B to protect yourself from future infection.

Co-infection with hepatitis C is common in people with human immunodeficiency virus (HIV); see Chapter 18 for information on dealing with this co-infection.

Chapter 3

Let's Get Ready to Rumble: Hepatitis C versus Your Immune System

*V*iruses are so small that you need a special microscope to see them. But size doesn't stop the hepatitis C virus from infecting the liver and creating havoc. After the virus infects, your immune system kicks in to try to fight the infection. Unfortunately, the body's immune system successfully eliminates only a small portion of hep C infections (about 15 to 25 percent). Most folks develop a chronic, or longer-term, infection that causes liver disease.

In this chapter, I fill you in on the mechanics of the hepatitis virus and how your body responds to it. I tell you what exactly hepatitis C virus is, what it does to trick the immune system, and why the immune system often fails to control the hep C infection.

Knowing what's going on with their body and disease at the smallest level appeals to many folks facing long-term illness. If you fall into this group, you'll dig this chapter. Others can take or leave some of the more technical-sounding info. If you fall into this group, you may want to simply skim over this chapter; that way, you'll at least know that the info is here, should you need it in the future.

When Viruses Attack

Virus infection (like hepatitis C infection, for example) starts off at a really tiny level, when a single virus infects a single cell. But from there, things quickly get out of control: Within hours, thousands of new viruses are formed from the one infected cell (see the "Tracking the Hepatitis C Virus Life Cycle" section, later in this chapter). Infection caused by even a small amount of virus multiplies quickly. Viruses can't multiply without the help of your cells.

The *cell* is the basis of all life — from the simple amoeba to a flower to your body. The human body has trillions of distinct *cells* that ultimately do things like digest your breakfast cereal or protect you from the cold virus going around town. Tiny cells get such large jobs done by working together. Cells work to form tissues, which work together to form organs, which work with other organs and cells to form systems (like your digestive and immune systems).

The cell of interest with hepatitis C is the liver cell. Millions of liver cells, or *hepatocytes,* make up the liver, which is one of the organs of the digestive system. But the liver also contributes to the immune, circulatory, and excretory systems. (For more information on the liver and liver cells, see Chapter 4.)

Picturing the hep C virus

So what's a virus, you may wonder. A *virus* is actually a small particle that infects cells. Biologists debate whether a virus is really alive because viruses can't live on their own. A virus must find a *host cell.* Unfortunately, your liver cells become the host for hep C virus.

The virus job description is straightforward: make more copies of itself (reproduce). Because they need to get into the host cell in order to reproduce, viruses have evolved tricky ways of entering the host cell and taking over to make more viruses.

Take a look at Figure 3-1 for an idea of what the hepatitis C virus looks like. Hepatitis C contains the basic viral components that all viruses have:

- ✔ **Viral genes:** Viral genes can come as DNA, like our own genes, or as a related nucleic acid called RNA. The hep C virus has RNA genes.

- ✔ **Viral capsid:** This protein coat (or shell) holds the viral genes (RNA for hep C). The capsid is sometimes called the *core protein.*

For more protection and to help them replicate, many viruses, including hepatitis C, also have the following:

- ✔ **Viral envelope:** This protein–lipid (fat) membrane surrounds the capsid and gives added protection. In the case of hepatitis C, the envelope is made of proteins called E1 and E2.

- ✔ **Viral enzymes:** Not shown in Figure 3-1 are the special enzymes made by the virus. Hep C doesn't carry these enzymes around, but makes them when it gets into your cells. Because viral enzymes are essential to the virus, many of them, such as *viral protease* (which breaks up viral protein into useable pieces), are targets for development of anti-hepatitis C drugs.

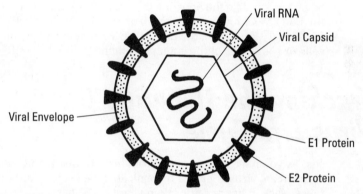

Figure 3-1: Hepatitis C virus.

Hitting the road to find host cells

Viral transmission is the way viruses move from one person to another. Viruses zip from one host to another in different ways. The following list contains some means of transmission for the different hepatitis viruses and the human immunodeficiency virus (HIV). For more information on the different types of hepatitis viruses and how hep C is transmitted, see Chapter 2.

- ✔ **Food or water contaminated with infected feces:** Hepatitis A and hepatitis E.

- ✔ **Blood from infected person:** Hepatitis B and hepatitis C and HIV. Because these three viruses share a route of transmission, it's possible to get more than one of these viruses.

- ✔ **Body fluids (semen, vaginal fluid, breast milk, and saliva) from infected person:** Hepatitis B and HIV. ***Note:*** Hepatitis C *is not* thought to be spread through body fluids, though it may be present.

Viruses are picky about their host species. A human virus won't want to live in a plant, or even a cat. And viruses have definite "room" or cell-type preferences within the body, as shown in these examples of different types of viruses:

- **Influenza viruses:** Respiratory tract
- **HIV:** T cells
- **Hepatitis virus:** Liver
- **Wart viruses (papilloma viruses):** Skin
- **Rabies virus:** Nerves

Some viruses, like the hepatitis C virus and HIV, infect other cells in the body too, though not as much as they infect their cell of choice. Preliminary studies on the hepatitis C virus show it may infect brain cells or some cells of the immune system.

Tracking the Hepatitis C Virus Life Cycle

Just as you have a cycle of life from birth to death and everything in between, viruses have a recognizable life cycle — although it takes place in hours rather than years.

Following the steps of cell infection

The following is a brief description of the stages of hepatitis C virus infection identified by scientists. (All viruses follow similar steps.) Follow along by using Figure 3-2.

1. **The hep C virus attaches to the liver cell.**

   Hep C attaches by recognizing and binding to one or more proteins on the cell surface, called *viral receptors,* which are normal cell proteins that the virus has evolved to use as its doorway into the cell.

2. **Hep C enters the liver cell.**

   After binding to its receptor, the virus crosses the cell membrane with the help of its receptor and moves into the liver cell, leaving its envelope outside as it enters.

3. Hep C "uncoats."

When hep C gets inside the cell, the first thing it does is take off its capsid (protein coat) so the viral RNA can get to business.

4. Hep C makes viral proteins and replicates RNA.

Hep C takes over the cells' machinery to make new virus proteins, including enzymes, the viral capsid, and the viral envelope. The enzymes help make copies of the RNA genes. This new RNA will be the viral genes for the newly created viruses. This step is called *replication*.

5. Hep C puts together new viruses.

Envelope, capsid, and RNA are assembled to make new hepatitis C viruses, a step known as hep C *reproduction*.

6. New hep C viruses exit the cell.

Newly released viruses may infect nearby liver cells or go into the blood. If you have hep C viruses in your blood, your viral RNA tests will be positive (see Chapter 6 for a discussion of viral tests).

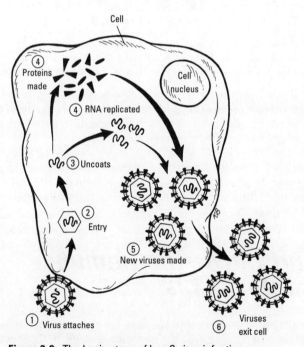

Figure 3-2: The basic steps of hep C virus infection.

Scientists have been hampered in studying the hep C viruses because growing hep C outside the body was difficult. New developments mean that more information about the nitty-gritty of hep C infection is being discovered, which helps in drug therapy development. The steps outlined above are intensely studied by researchers who are looking for ways to block one of these steps.

Changing the virus genes

The hepatitis C virus is so successful at staying in your body because it can subtly change its genes. (These subtle changes are called *mutations.*) This little devil of a virus has figured out how to escape from your body's normal ways of attacking it (see the "Fighting Back: The Immune System Responds" section, later in this chapter).

Because of all this changing around, hep C viruses aren't exactly the same from person to person. Here's a list of the types of variations scientists find in the hepatitis C virus:

- ✓ A *genotype* is a distinct group of a hepatitis virus. Six different genotypes have been identified, which I describe in Chapter 6. They're called genotypes 1 through 6.

- ✓ A *subtype* is a subdivision among different genotypes. There are at least 30 different subtypes of hepatitis C. For example, genotype 1a and genotype 1b are subtypes of genotype 1.

- ✓ If you hear the term *quasispecies,* don't get frightened. The term just means that within any batch of virus, there are lots of slightly different viruses, but these differences are too slight to be called a genotype or subtype.

Hepatitis C virus may use these changes in virus genes to stay alive despite attack from the immune system or antiviral drugs. For example, certain genotypes are more resistant to drug treatment (see Chapter 8).

Fighting Back: The Immune System Responds

Now I'm going to delve into the *immune system,* which is what your body uses to fight against the hepatitis C virus. In this section, I describe some of the basics and try to explain why the human immune system doesn't always work against hepatitis C (scientists are still figuring that one out). It's also important to recognize that your immune system actually causes much of the disease with hepatitis C.

The immune system protects you by detecting and destroying "foreigners," such as viruses and cancer cells. As with many wars, the immune system's fight against infection can seem like an endless battle, with fatalities on both sides. The immune system uses an intricate network of cells and proteins that work together to form the *immune response.* When you're protected from a foreign agent, you're said to be *immune,* or to have *immunity* from that foreign agent.

Immunization and *vaccination* mean the same thing and refer to the procedure whereby pieces of a foreign agent *(antigen)* are introduced to your immune system in the hope of inducing long-lasting immunity. Of the hepatitis viruses, vaccines are available only for hepatitis A and hepatitis B.

Getting to know the players

The immune system uses organs such as the thymus and spleen, as well as tissues in your lymph nodes, bone marrow, liver, and intestines. But the major players are cells and molecules, which I now describe:

- **Antigen:** Small segments on each "foreigner" (called *antigens*) are recognized by the immune system. Antigens are part of the signal for the immune system to attack. The hepatitis C virus has multiple antigens.

- **T and B cells (lymphocyte):** These are the cells that go after antigen. Each lymphocyte recognizes one specific antigen out of the millions of possible antigens it could run up against. Here are the background and job description for these important cells:

  - **B cells** mature in the bone marrow, which is the spongy inside part of bones. They make *antibodies,* which are Y-shaped proteins that bind to antigen. Another name for antibody is *immunoglobulin.*

  - **T cells** mature in the thymus, which is located underneath the ribs high in the chest. Two types of T cells are: the T helper cell, which helps B cells make antibody, and the T killer cell, which directly kills virus-infected cells.

✔ **Cytokines:** Messenger proteins that signal other cells of the immune system or other cells in the body. Interferon, used as a drug to kill hepatitis C virus, is one type of cytokine. Cytokines can be made by any white blood cell, whether specific for antigen or not.

See Figure 3-3 for an idea of how these players fit together to give an immune response that is specific to hepatitis C antigen. When the virus is inside of your liver cells, T killer cells attack during what's called a *cell-mediated immune response*. When the virus is roaming your body on its own, the *antibody-mediated immune response* sends antibody to bind to the virus to keep it from infecting your cells.

There's also another part of the immune response, called the *innate response,* that uses cytokines and white blood cells to fight against hepatitis C. Scientists are researching both of these types of immune responses — specific and innate — to learn why some people can eliminate hepatitis C virus on their own and others do not.

Because the immune system must do its work all over the body, or wherever a virus might be, the cells and molecules of the immune response must be able to move around and get together, which they do through the blood and lymph.

Cell Mediated Immune Response

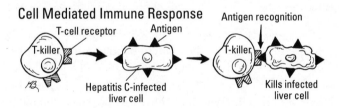

Antibody Mediated Immune Response

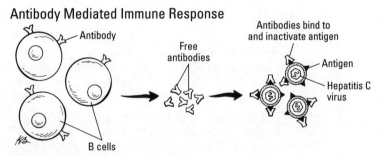

Figure 3-3: The specific immune response to hepatitis C virus.

Examining the blood

Blood is a mixture of cells and liquid that travels through your arteries and veins, pumped by the heart. The components of blood include:

- **Red blood cells (RBC):** The RBC carry oxygen through the body.

- **White blood cells (WBC):** These agents of the immune response include lymphocytes, monocytes, neutrophils, eosinophils, and basophils. If you have a WBC count performed on your blood (see Chapter 7), the levels of each of these cells are tested.

- **Platelets:** They help in blood clotting.

- **Plasma:** Cells float in this liquid (also called *serum*), which contains nutrients and proteins like albumin and fibrinogen, which are both made by the liver (see Chapter 4), and *antibodies* that circulate to protect you against infection.

I talk about blood throughout the book. Hepatitis C is transmitted through blood; if you have hep C, you'll have lots of blood tests; when you're on drug treatment, you'll be checked for problems with your blood (anemia); and blood-clotting problems can arise with cirrhosis. If you want to know more about blood, check out an educational course on blood (hematology) put on the Web by the Puget Sound Blood Center (www.psbc.org/education/hematology).

Describing lymph

Lymph is a clear liquid that moves through a special circulatory system of lymphatic vessels and bathes tissues of the body. Lymph vessels pass through strategic tissues and organs, including your lymph nodes, spleen, liver, and intestines (see Figure 3-4).

The purpose of the lymph system is to bring together antigen and cells of the immune system. The lymph nodes are a meeting place for the immune system to launch its attack.

Battling the hep C infection

The hep C virus and your immune system each do their best to win the battle of infection. Hep C wants to stay in your body. Your immune system wants hep C to leave. Hep C mutates to avoid your immune system (see the section "Changing the virus genes," earlier in this chapter).

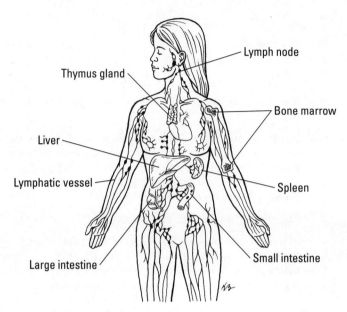

Figure 3-4: The lymphatic system.

The immune system reacts to hep C infection by increasing blood flow, bringing in white blood cells, and closing off the infected area, all in the effort to control the infection and prevent its spread. These defensive actions cause inflammation of the liver. For most folks with hep C, inflammation doesn't appear to control the infection; rather, it actually damages the liver cells.

The damage caused by temporary inflammation can be reversed. When inflammation continues, however, the liver replaces its damaged cells with scar tissue (fibrosis). Continued scarring leads to cirrhosis or irreversible liver damage.

Your immune response, which is supposed to protect you from hep C infection, may thus — in its overly zealous but ultimately misguided response — contribute to liver disease. The goal of medical treatment against hep C is to help the body fight hep C infection so that inflammation stops.

You can keep your immune system in tip-top shape by eating well, avoiding toxins, and staying calm — advice that I discuss in Part III.

Chapter 4

Infecting the Liver: Symptoms and Progression of the Disease

In This Chapter
▶ Describing the liver and its functions
▶ Understanding hep C symptoms
▶ Seeing how the disease progresses

*Y*our liver is an essential organ. Sitting in the center of your body, the liver processes the food you eat and eliminates poisons. When hepatitis C infects liver cells, any of the liver's hundreds of functions can be affected.

Hepatitis C symptoms let you know your body needs help. You may have symptoms that range from none or annoying to serious or life-threatening. Treatment in the early stages of hep C can protect you from developing liver failure or liver cancer (see Chapters 8 and 10). If treatment doesn't work, or if you find out about your hep C at a later stage, you still have options for your healthcare and lifestyle that can improve your symptoms and quality of life (see Part III). In this chapter, I give you basic information about the liver and hepatitis C disease.

Looking at Your Liver

The liver is a powerhouse of an organ, performing its jobs 24 hours a day, 7 days a week. When you find out you have hepatitis C and start experiencing symptoms as a result of your liver infection, you're going to want to know all you can about this essential organ.

Mapping it out

The human liver weighs in at a smooth 3 pounds and is about the size of a football, making it your biggest internal organ. To visualize its shape, you could take a trip to a supermarket and look at some animal livers in the meat department. Or a much simpler avenue of exploration is to check out Figure 4-1.

You can't really feel your liver by poking at your torso, because it's located under the bottom of the rib cage — on the right side, under the diaphragm. Your stomach and spleen are next door to your liver, and the gallbladder, small intestine, and right kidney are just beneath it.

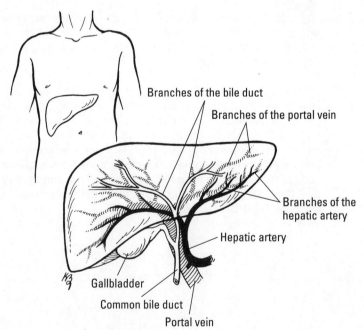

Figure 4-1: Looking closely at your liver.

Your liver is filled with blood, fed by the *portal vein* (which delivers nutritious blood from the digestive tract) and the *hepatic artery* (which brings oxygenated blood from the heart).

In addition to all the blood vessels in the liver, there are vessels for the *biliary system,* which is made up of bile ducts and the gallbladder. One function of the biliary system is to drain the liver of waste products by way of the bile ducts. The liver makes *bile,* which is a thick greenish fluid that contains bile salts, cholesterol, and liver waste. Bile goes to your gallbladder, which acts as a storage area. When you eat a meal, the second main function of the biliary system kicks in. Bile is sent from the gallbladder to the small intestine so that the bile salts can be used to digest the fats you eat. Bile, carrying the liver's waste products, leaves the intestines through the feces and is responsible for the brown color of feces.

De-livering function

The liver is a master organ, performing more than 500 essential jobs. When hep C causes liver damage, any of the following tasks of the liver may be affected. The more serious the damage by hep C, as in cirrhosis, the more serious the effect will be on liver function (see the section "Cirrhosis," later in this chapter). In the following sections, I group the liver's 500-plus jobs into four main categories.

Processing plant

Most things you ingest, be they food or medications, need to be processed into forms that the body can use. Two examples are:

- ✔ Carbohydrates from food are turned into *glucose* (a form of sugar) for instant energy, and then glucose is converted to glycogen for storage. When blood sugar levels drop, glycogen is converted back to glucose.

- ✔ Normal processing of protein in the body leads to production of ammonia. The liver takes the toxic ammonia and converts it to urea, which is then eliminated in urine.

Production facility

The liver is like a production factory, making hormones, proteins, and other substances essential to the body.

Here's a list of some of the proteins made by the liver. Your doctor can test your blood for these proteins, and when levels are low, this is an indicator of liver impairment (see Chapter 7).

- ✔ **Albumin:** This is the major protein in the blood. When the liver is impaired, albumin levels drop. Low albumin levels may contribute to the problem of edema, or swelling.

✔ **Enzymes:** Alanine aminotransferase (ALT) and other enzymes (see Chapter 7) are used by the liver to convert substances to usable forms.

✔ **Blood-clotting proteins:** You need these proteins so you don't bleed to death. One of these proteins is called *prothrombin,* and the *prothrombin time* test (called *PT*) measures how long it takes your blood to clot.

But the liver production process isn't limited to proteins. It also produces other molecules, such as *cholesterol.* In fact, the liver makes 85 percent of all cholesterol, and cholesterol is necessary for the body to make sex hormones, bile salts, and vitamin D.

The liver makes *bile,* a fluid that moves through the biliary system, described in the section "Looking at Your Liver," earlier in this chapter. Bile helps your body use fats and vitamins, and breaks down excess cholesterol. When the liver is damaged, bile builds up in the body, and the bilirubin causes the yellow coloring of jaundice. Chapter 7 discusses tests for bilirubin.

Storage space and filtration system

The liver is a warehouse, and within its cells, essential nutrients are stored that are released when needed. Sugar is stored as glycogen for energy, and the liver also stores vitamins and minerals — vitamin A and iron, for example.

The liver also filters toxic waste that reaches it from the blood and also the waste it creates as it processes substances. Toxins (poisons) are then sent out of the body through urine or feces.

Experiencing Symptoms

Symptoms are the body's way of telling you to pay attention. If you have hep C virus, you may be *asymptomatic,* meaning that you have no symptoms at all, or you may have symptoms that are mild or initially confused with other illnesses.

Soon after you first become infected with the hep C virus, you may have flu-like symptoms or even *jaundice* (abnormally yellow skin or eyes) during the *acute phase* (within the first six months) of infection. Most people in the acute phase don't notice any symptoms.

When your disease becomes *chronic* (after six months), you may develop some of the following symptoms in the months or even decades after infection.

You probably won't have all of these symptoms, but being aware of possible symptoms is good, so if one of them does occur, you'll recognize it. Keep in mind that some symptoms happen as a function of aging, stress, or menopause. And as I mention throughout the book, each person with hepatitis C is an individual, and your symptoms depend on so many factors.

- ✔ **Fatigue:** In a class of its own, the most commonly reported symptom

- ✔ **Digestive problems:** Nausea, vomiting, diarrhea, bloating, gas, indigestion, abdominal pain, loss of appetite

- ✔ **Emotional problems:** Depression, anxiety, mood swings

- ✔ **Flu-like symptoms:** Headache, low-grade fever, night sweats, chills, joint and muscle pain, weakness

- ✔ **Hormonal problems:** More intense premenstrual tension or menopausal symptoms, irregular periods, loss of sex drive, erectile dysfunction

- ✔ **Jaundice:** Yellowing of skin or eyes, dark urine, pale or clay-colored stools

- ✔ **Skin problems:** Dry skin, itchy skin, bruising, reddened palms, red spidery spots, swelling of your hands, feet, or face

- ✔ **Sleep problems:** Insomnia, night sweats

- ✔ **Thinking problems:** Brain fog, *encephalopathy* (severe brain problems with cirrhosis)

I list some more specific symptoms of cirrhosis and end stage liver diseases in the corresponding sections for these conditions later in the chapter.

Your hep C may directly cause some symptoms; others may be side effects of medications or the result of worrying about your illness. Like the chicken and the egg, it doesn't matter what came first. If you have symptoms as described above, or any others, tell your physician. Working with your doctor, you can deal with your symptoms. (I cover the treatment options and tips for working with your doctor in Part II.)

Now — today — is the time to implement changes in your diet and lifestyle that will help you deal with some of these symptoms. Trying the mind-body therapies and light exercise described in Chapter 13 may reduce stress and ease symptoms like insomnia, anxiety, and fatigue. Eating well and avoiding fried foods can help with many of the gastrointestinal problems (see Chapter 11 for more on nutrition). Your support group also may have tips for dealing with the symptoms of hep C (see Chapter 14). You need not suffer — and certainly not in silence!

Describing the Progression of Hepatitis C

Hepatitis C virus infection is classified into two distinct phases: acute and chronic. What distinguishes hepatitis C from other hepatitis viruses (see Chapter 2) is the fact that the virus infection becomes chronic in about 75 to 85 percent of folks infected. See Figure 4-2 for a representation of hepatitis C disease progression that I cover in this section.

The acute phase

The time period up to six months after you're infected with the hepatitis C virus is called the *acute* phase of hep C disease. At this point, many people don't know they're infected, but some folks experience flu-like symptoms (such as fever, aches, and tiredness) or jaundice-related symptoms (such as yellowing skin, dark urine, and light stools).

A rare complication during acute infection is called *fulminant hepatic failure,* which means liver failure and requires emergency medical attention.

If you clear (or get rid of) the virus at this stage, you won't develop the chronic phase of hep C, described in the following section. About 15 to 25 percent of people infected are able to stop the virus in its tracks during the acute phase. But the majority of people go on to have a chronic infection. Researchers are studying why some people launch an immune response that can successfully block hep C. (I cover the immune response to hepatitis C in Chapter 3.)

If you've successfully eliminated hepatitis C virus, you'll still make antibodies to hep C and have a positive hep C antibody test (see Chapter 6 for more details). Your RNA test (the test that tells you if hepatitis C virus is currently present) will be negative, and your antibodies will probably not protect you from future infection with hepatitis C, so take precautions not to get reinfected.

The chronic phase

At six months and more after infection, your disease is considered to be chronic. Approximately 75 to 85 percent of people with hepatitis C develop chronic infection. I outline the possible phases of chronic hepatitis C in Figure 4-2 and describe them in the next sections in order of progression — from no liver damage to inflammation, fibrosis, cirrhosis, or end stage liver disease.

The following factors have been shown to contribute to more severe disease progression:

- ✔ Being over 40 at the time of infection
- ✔ Being male
- ✔ Drinking alcohol
- ✔ Being co-infected with hepatitis B or HIV
- ✔ Having fatty liver disease (see Chapter 11)

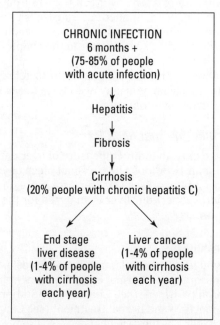

CHRONIC INFECTION
6 months +
(75-85% of people
with acute infection)

↓

Hepatitis

↓

Fibrosis

↓

Cirrhosis
(20% people with chronic hepatitis C)

End stage
liver disease
(1-4% of people
with cirrhosis
each year)

Liver cancer
(1-4% of people
with cirrhosis
each year)

Figure 4-2: The progression of chronic hepatitis C disease.

You can't change the fact that you're over 40, you're a man, or you're already infected with hepatitis B or HIV. But you can avoid getting infected with these viruses (see Chapter 2 for a discussion of transmission through blood or body fluids). And stopping drinking is probably the single most important change you can make to save your liver (see Chapter 12).

Liver cancer is a complication that can occur when you have cirrhosis. And diseases outside the liver can also develop with hepatitis C virus. I cover these conditions later in the chapter.

Inflammation and fibrosis

The earliest phase of hep C disease is liver inflammation. (*Hepatitis* literally means inflammation of the liver.) Inflammation occurs when immune cells enter the liver to kill the hep C virus. The fight put up by the immune cells damages liver cells (see Chapter 2).

If unstopped, over a period of time, the inflammation can turn into scarring, which is called *fibrosis*. The liver can recover from inflammation and minor scarring, but continued scarring leads to problems with liver function and possibly irreversible scarring, which is called *cirrhosis* (see the corresponding section later in the chapter).

If you have inflammation or fibrosis, it's important to get regular monitoring from your physician; you may need tests to see whether you're slipping into further liver damage.

How do you know whether you have it?

Liver enzyme tests are only an indirect measure of liver damage. To directly see what your liver looks like, a small piece of your liver is examined from a biopsy (see Chapter 7 for more on liver tests). Under the microscope, your liver is analyzed for the degree of inflammation or fibrosis.

What can you do about it?

If you find out that you have liver inflammation or fibrosis, stay calm, and review your options. Pharmaceutical treatment involves combination interferon treatment (see Chapter 8). Additional options include acupuncture and herbal treatment (see Chapter 10), diet changes (see Chapter 11), lifestyle changes (see Chapter 13), and a positive outlook (see Chapter 14).

Cirrhosis

When fibrosis becomes extensive over the whole liver, you have cirrhosis. Around 20 percent of people with chronic hepatitis C get cirrhosis of the liver after decades of infection. Cirrhosis was called *irreversible liver scarring* in the past, but it's now thought that early stages of cirrhosis may be reversible. Cirrhosis is called *compensated* if the normal liver cells make up for the damage. When cirrhosis is *decompensated,* your liver is starting to fail (see the next section on liver failure).

With cirrhosis, you may have the following symptoms:

- ✔ Ascites (buildup of fluid in the abdomen)
- ✔ Swelling of the legs
- ✔ Small red blood vessels on the skin
- ✔ Bleeding hemorrhoids
- ✔ Decreased urination
- ✔ Nosebleed or bleeding gums
- ✔ Breast development in men
- ✔ Severe itching (buildup of uncleared toxins)
- ✔ Bone loss

Symptoms of cirrhosis can become life-threatening as cirrhosis develops into liver failure. If you're vomiting blood or experiencing chest pains, get emergency medical care.

How do you know whether you have it?

Abnormal results of liver tests can point to cirrhosis, especially in decompensated cirrhosis. Tests of albumin, bleeding times (prothrombin), and bilirubin tell a lot about how your liver is functioning. A biopsy reveals the extent of damage to your liver.

What can you do about it?

If you have compensated cirrhosis, consider more aggressive treatment for your hep C, if you haven't already done so. Don't drink alcohol, and do everything you can to save your liver — and your life. For decompensated cirrhosis, see the next section, "Liver failure."

When you have cirrhosis, it's important to get tested regularly for liver cancer and liver function.

Liver failure

Continuing cirrhosis can lead to liver failure. *End-stage liver disease* (ESLD) and *decompensated cirrhosis* are ways of describing irreversible scarring that keeps the liver from functioning, a condition known as *liver failure*. About 20 percent of people with cirrhosis develop end stage liver disease. The following can result from liver failure:

- ✔ **Portal hypertension:** Within a scarred liver, blood can't flow normally, which results in portal hypertension. Your portal vein (see Figure 4-1), which normally carries blood to the liver, gets slowed down, and pressure inside the vein increases. Higher blood pressure (hypertension) in the portal vein is called *portal hypertension*. Because other blood vessels must take blood back to the heart, they become swollen due to increased blood flow, resulting in what's called *varices,* or thin walls in blood vessels that can easily break and bleed, which you may experience as vomiting blood.

- ✔ **Ascites:** This condition results from fluid buildup in your abdominal cavity. Ascites are a complication of portal hypertension and other factors. They're treated with diuretics and other medications. To help alleviate the condition, avoid salty foods (see Chapter 11).

- ✔ **Encephalopathy:** Brain and nervous system damage can result from liver failure. You may have problems with reflexes, personality changes, or loss of consciousness.

How do you know whether you have it?

Different blood tests (albumin, prothrombin time, and bilirubin) indicate the seriousness of your illness. At this stage, the symptoms are so obvious that a doctor who is knowledgeable about liver disease will immediately recognize the severity of your disease.

What can you do about it?

Stay calm, and get referred for a liver transplant (see Chapter 9). While waiting for a new liver, watching your diet and lifestyle is especially important.

Liver cancer

Hepatocellular carcinoma (HCC), or hepatoma, is more common in other parts of the world and occurs mainly with hepatitis virus B or C in Canada and the United States. HCC is a primary liver cancer, meaning that it develops in the liver and isn't a secondary cancer that moves to the liver from elsewhere in the body (called *metastasis*). Between 1 and 4 percent of people with cirrhosis develop liver cancer each year.

How do you know whether you have it?

If you have cirrhosis, you should be monitored for development of liver cancer. A blood test called alpha-fetoprotein can detect cancer in some people. Liver scans and biopsies are used to detect tumors (see Chapter 7). Speak to your doctor about having regular scans if you have cirrhosis.

What can you do about it?

Early-stage liver cancer is easier to treat with surgery than later-stage cancer. *Resection surgery,* in which the liver tumors are removed, or *transplant surgery,* in which the liver is entirely replaced, can both be performed. Transplant surgery has a better longer-term success rate, but donor livers are in short supply. (See Chapter 9 for more on transplants.) For later-stage cancer, drug treatment trials are an option (see Chapter 8 for some information on clinical trials).

Diseases outside the liver

Illnesses that aren't directly due to liver damage are called *extra-hepatic* manifestations of hep C infection. About 1 or 2 percent of people with hepatitis C virus get these extrahepatic diseases.

In the process of fighting the hep C virus, your body produces antibodies that might hurt the body by causing autoimmune reactions, which means fighting the body, or an accumulation of antibody to such a degree that it "clogs up" parts of the body. The following are thought to be caused by the immune response to hep C infection:

- ✔ **Cryoglobulinemia:** Results from the buildup of clumps of hepatitis C virus bound to antibody *(antibody complexes)*. These antibody complexes can affect the skin, joints, kidneys, and nerves. The name *cryo* means *cold,* and *globulin* is *antibody.* In the laboratory, these antibodies clump up in the cold.

- ✔ **Glomerulonephritis:** Kidney inflammation caused by the antibody complexes being deposited in the internal structures of the kidney *(glomeruli)*, causing an inflammation of the kidney.

Another type of extrahepatic disease caused by hep C is *porphyria cutanea tarda* (PCT). This illness occurs because the liver isn't making a particular enzyme, and it can lead to blistering in areas of the skin exposed to sunlight. To learn more about PCT, check out www.porphyriafoundation.com.

Scientists are studying whether other diseases, such as thyroid disorders and *lichen planus,* a disorder of the skin, are caused by hep C. Hep C may possibly infect other types of cells in addition to liver cells, which may cause certain symptoms of hepatitis C or contribute to other diseases. Research is ongoing to see which other illnesses are linked to hep C.

How do you know whether you have it?

New symptoms, such as problems with your skin or urination, can alert your doctor to a problem. There are specific blood tests for cryoglobulins. An examination of your urine or a kidney biopsy can check for glomerulonephritis. PCT can be determined by testing your urine and blood.

What can you do about it?

Interferon or steroids may be helpful in treating these illnesses. See your doctor to discuss treatment options. Drug treatment for hepatitis C (see Chapter 8) may also be helpful in treating extrahepatic diseases.

Part II
Diagnosing and Treating the Disease

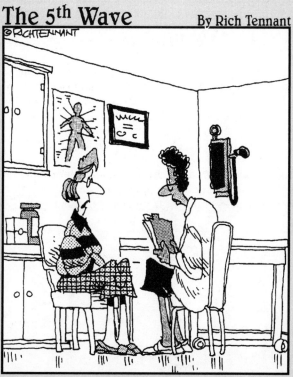

"Actually, I didn't experience any itching until after I started inhaling the scent strips in the waiting room magazines."

In this part . . .

You'll probably see a variety of healthcare professionals during your journey with hep C. Regular laboratory tests for hepatitis C virus and liver function determine how far your disease has progressed and help plan the right treatment. You may choose to try combination peginterferon plus ribavirin, which is successful in approximately half or more of all people treated, though serious side effects can occur. Other health approaches include alternative treatments, such as acupuncture and herbs. I cover all of these issues and liver transplants in this part.

Chapter 5

Building Your Medical Support Team

The keys to an excellent support system start with you and your healthcare providers. You need to have a medical doctor experienced in hepatitis C to lead you through the maze of tests, guide you to the best treatment available, and support you in your healthcare decisions.

As in all relationships, the doctor-patient interaction demands good communication from both parties. Your doctor needs to keep you well informed about your hepatitis C and answer your questions. Your job is to tell your doctor about your symptoms; concerns; and any medications, herbs, or supplements you take.

In this chapter, I discuss choosing, communicating with, and working with your doctor and other healthcare providers. I also provide some ideas on keeping records of your hepatitis C tests and treatments in a special notebook, to make all that communication easier.

Starting with Your Primary Care Provider

For many people, the primary care provider (PCP) is the point of entry into the healthcare system. And it's at this point of entry, while working with their PCP, that millions of folks have discovered that they have hepatitis C.

The healthcare practitioner whom you visit for your routine physical examination is your PCP. Primary care provides long-term care that includes prevention, finding and treating common medical problems, and referring you to medical specialists. Many health plans require that you visit a PCP before going to a specialist (see Chapter 16 to read about health insurance and the "Moving on to Specialists" section, later in this chapter, for more on hepatitis C specialists).

Most PCPs are physicians (another term for medical doctor), with one of these degrees and titles:

- **Medical doctor (MD):** Training includes four years of medical school and three to seven years of *residency* training (in which the first year may be called an internship) in a chosen specialty, such as family medicine, obstetrics and gynecology, or internal medicine.

  Some doctors further train for a *fellowship* in their specialty or subspecialty (such as gastroenterology as a subspecialty of internal medicine).

- **Doctor of osteopathy (DO):** The DO and MD degrees are identical, except that the DO degree includes additional topics on manipulation of bones and muscles. Doctors of osteopathy attend a school of osteopathic medicine, rather than a school of medicine, for the first four years of medical training.

  DOs undergo identical residency and fellowship training as MDs. About 5 percent of all doctors in America are doctors of osteopathy.

Two other types of healthcare practitioners can serve as primary care providers:

- **Nurse practitioner (NP):** Registered nurses (RNs) with master's-level training who work with physicians or in solo practice.

- **Physician assistant (PA):** These folks receive basic medical training (26 months) and work alongside physicians to provide healthcare.

When NPs and PAs become *certified* by passing a national exam, they might use the term NP-C or PA-C after their name, with the *C* indicating their certification. Both NPs and PAs can specialize or receive additional training in their fields. The requirements for NPs and PAs vary by specialty and location, so check with your individual health providers, insurance plans, and state regulations for more information.

Within primary care, some doctors specialize in treating different types of people. You may visit a different practitioner depending on your age or gender. The following are the general categories for doctors, but your NP or PA might also fit into one of the PCP specialties.

- ✔ **General practitioners:** These doctors provide healthcare for a wide range of medical problems. They don't focus on any special areas of medicine.

- ✔ **Family practitioners:** These physicians are similar to general practitioners, but they have additional training to focus on healthcare for family members of all ages, including children.

- ✔ **Obstetrician/gynecologists:** Women may use these doctors as their PCP, especially women of childbearing age.

- ✔ **Pediatricians:** These doctors care for infants, children, and adolescents.

- ✔ **Internists:** These doctors care for adults.

Pediatricians and internists may specialize and treat specific parts of the body or specific diseases, in which case they become specialists (for example, a cardiologist or gastroenterologist).

 You may wonder how to interpret your doctor's credentials. All doctors (MDs and DOs) are licensed to practice medicine by their individual states. *Board certification* is an additional qualification that means the doctor has completed residency training and completed exams in one of the 24 medical specialties, such as internal medicine or family medicine.

 After your diagnosis with hepatitis C, your PCP will most likely refer you to a liver specialist, who has experience in treating hepatitis C. The liver specialist performs further testing and treatment for your hepatitis C and communicates results with your PCP. Your PCP remains your point of reference for health issues not related to hepatitis C and is the guardian of your overall healthcare.

Moving on to Specialists

Medicine has become a specialized business, with an almost overwhelming amount of information available today on different parts of the body. It's impossible for any one doctor to be an expert in every area of medicine. Consequently, when you have hepatitis C, you want a doctor with the most up-to-date knowledge of and experience with hep C.

Hepatitis C virus primarily causes liver disease, so you're looking for a doctor who knows the liver (and hep C) inside out. The physician specialists who treat hepatitis C may be called one of the following:

- ✓ **Gastroenterologists:** Specializing in the many diseases of the digestive tract, gastroenterologists vary in the amount of experience they have with liver diseases or hepatitis C. You may see the letters *GI* in connection with gastroenterologists, which comes from the term *gastrointestinal.*

- ✓ **Hepatologists:** These doctors are liver specialists who in many cases are also gastroenterologists.

- ✓ **Infectious-disease specialists:** Hepatitis C is a virus infection, so you might be referred to an infectious-disease doctor. Some infectious-disease specialists have experience treating hepatitis C.

Most people with hepatitis C visit a gastroenterologist or hepatologist, but some folks, especially those with an HIV co-infection, may go to an infectious-disease doctor who has expertise in hepatitis C treatment.

 Specialist doctors spend many years learning their trade. Gastroenterologists who treat adults first specialize in internal medicine (residency) and then get training in gastroenterology (additional residency). Pediatric gastroenterologists first specialize in pediatrics (residency) and then in gastroenterology (additional residency). A *residency* is a period of hospital-based training in a medical specialty after the basic four years of medical school.

Because gastroenterology is such a large field (read about how large the digestive system is in Chapter 11), different residency programs vary in how much time they devote to liver diseases or hepatitis C. Some doctors take additional training, called a fellowship, in hepatology, which is specific training in liver diseases. A *fellowship* is the name for another period of hospital-based training that usually occurs after the years of residency training.

In this chapter and much of the book, I focus on treatment by gastroenterologists/hepatologists. You may also find NPs and PAs with specialist hepatology training. The American Association for the Study of Liver Disease has a training fellowship for NPs and PAs.

Reviewing the job description

Your liver specialist will apply his expert knowledge to treat your hepatitis C, using the three-pronged approach used by all health-care professionals:

- ✔ **Diagnosis:** Your doctor notes your symptoms and your general physical appearance and uses up-to-date techniques to test your liver and overall health. Blood tests, sonograms or CT scans, and liver biopsies (which I cover in Chapters 6 and 7) are among the laboratory tools your doctor uses to arrive at a diagnosis.

- ✔ **Treatment:** Using the most effective and safest medications, your doctor will treat your hepatitis C and also any side effects resulting from hepatitis C disease or hepatitis C drug treatment. I cover drug treatment for hepatitis C in Chapter 8.

- ✔ **Management:** Your doctor manages your health over a long period of time by seeing you during office visits and ordering laboratory tests. Sometimes, management of your hepatitis C involves referring you to other healthcare providers. For example, your doctor may refer you to a psychiatrist if she suspects that you may be suffering from depression.

Finding qualified candidates

Check your health insurance policy to find out its rules about visiting specialists. With some health plans, you need a referral from your PCP, and some plans may limit your choice to doctors in their network or on their preferred-provider list. (But you can always telephone or write a letter to try to get access to an out-of-plan liver specialist if none is available on your plan.)

Doctors specializing in all things liver can be tricky to find. Many health insurance companies don't list hepatologists as a type of specialist. Hepatology is usually listed under gastroenterology, and you have to check with each gastroenterologist individually to see whether he has experience with hepatitis C. Here are some tips for finding a specialist to treat your hepatitis C:

- ✔ Your PCP is the first source for information on finding a specialist. Your other doctors and healthcare professionals may also provide referrals.

- ✔ The American Liver Foundation (ALF) (phone 800-465-4837; Web site www.liverfoundation.org) or Hepatitis Foundation

> International (phone 800-891-0707; Web site www.hepfi.org) can help you find a gastroenterologist or hepatologist in your area.
>
> ✔ Your state medical association can provide names of specialists. Look in your phone book for the telephone number.
>
> ✔ Local hospitals have lists of specialists.
>
> ✔ Local support groups of people with hepatitis C in your area can recommend doctors and give you tips on what to look for (see Chapter 14).

Examining the Doctor-Patient Relationship

The reality of healthcare today is that the patient — you — must be his or her own best advocate. The fact that you're reading this book shows your concern and desire to be an informed healthcare participant.

After you find one or more potential specialists (see the earlier section "Moving on to Specialists"), consider requesting an appointment to "interview" these doctors. You can then ask specific questions that will give both you and the practitioner a chance to see how well you agree on the treatment and management of your hepatitis C.

Getting to know your preferences

Healthcare decisions are a matter of personal choice, and people are as different as snowflakes. Knowing what's most important to you will help you obtain the healthcare you need. You have to decide what you're willing to do and put up with to get well. Can you conscientiously and consistently take your medication (see Chapter 8)? Do you favor Chinese medicine and other integrative approaches (see Chapter 10)? Are you willing to pursue a variety of self-help techniques (discussed in Part III)? Answering questions such as these are an important first step in making healthcare choices.

Treating and managing your hepatitis C should be a collaborative process. But psychic abilities aren't a prerequisite for other members of the team; you have to know yourself so you can communicate your questions, preferences, and concerns.

Think about previous healthcare experiences you've had. What did you like or dislike? Here's a list of things to consider. Your doctor may ask you about some of these things.

What types of health insurance and emotional support do you have?

✔ **What's your healthcare insurance situation?** Read your policy and make inquiries before you visit your doctor. See Chapter 16 for information on financial issues and health insurance.

✔ **Do you have a personal support system?** What will you do if you need help or a shoulder to lean on? Talk to family members, friends, and co-workers. See Chapter 14 for information on finding the support you need.

✔ **Do you belong to a support group?** Your doctor may encourage you to get this help from other people with hepatitis C because they're well prepared to help you on this journey.

Can you communicate your healthcare style — the types of issues that are important to you — to your doctor?

✔ **Are you the type of person who avoids all drugs unless absolutely necessary?** Your doctor needs to know whether you mind taking drugs so that he can best treat your hep C and any side effects.

✔ **Do you want to be a vocal partner in your healthcare?** Let your doctor know that you need to be actively involved in making decisions.

✔ **Do you use alternative or complementary medicine?** Doctors vary widely in their knowledge and support of alternative and complementary medicine. Your role as patient is to communicate with your doctor and educate him about complementary and alternative medicine (CAM), if need be.

How honest will you be with your doctor? Are you willing to make changes to your lifestyle?

✔ **Will you be honest about your current or former use of alcohol or recreational drugs?** If you currently smoke, drink, or use drugs (see Chapter 12 for a discussion of these dangerous substances), you also need to seriously consider whether you're willing to work with your doctor to go into treatment or follow up on a referral to an addiction counselor, if necessary.

- ✔ **Will you be conscientious about tracking your use of medications, drugs, herbs, and vitamins?** If you use these substances, will you write them down and tell your doctor that you're using them?

- ✔ **Will you talk about your concerns about sex?** It's possible for hepatitis C to be spread through sexual activity that involves exposure to blood. You may have concerns about transmission or about interest in sex, which can decrease as a side effect of hep C or drug treatment.

- ✔ **Will you change your diet or exercise routine to help your hep C symptoms?** Not all hepatitis C patients can or will alter their lifestyle.

When you find a doctor with whom you're comfortable, you're more likely to talk about the things that are really important to you, thus enabling your doctor to give you the best care.

Getting to know your doctor

Doctors vary in their experience with hepatitis C and their outlook on the disease. A doctor who has treated many different people with hepatitis C and is active in research can use his breadth of experience and resources to help you get well. But just because a doctor has lots of experience with hepatitis C doesn't mean he's the best doctor for *you.*

Use the following questions to think about what's important to look for in a prospective doctor or to better understand your current doctor. I can't give you the right answers because the best doctor for you probably has different answers than the best doctor for someone else.

You won't want to use all of these questions — not in the first visit, anyway — but they do give you an idea of things to look for. If you feel intimidated by the idea of asking the doctor anything, just pick a couple of the most relevant questions. You can also ask some questions of nurses or administrators in the office.

Find out your doctor's training and experience with hep C by asking some or all of these questions:

- ✔ **What specific training have you had in hepatitis C or liver disease?** Find out whether the doctor has had fellowship training (see the "Moving on to Specialists" section, earlier in the chapter) or other experience in liver disease.

✔ **How do you keep up to date about new information on hepatitis C?** Ask the doctor what professional publications he reads and whether he attends medical conferences on hepatitis C.

✔ **What's your personal experience with hepatitis C?** Ask how long the doctor has been treating people with hep C and how many people he treats in a year.

✔ **How much experience have you had with liver biopsies?** Ask the doctor how many liver biopsies he performs each year. You might also ask how long the doctor has been performing liver biopsies, which I discuss in Chapter 7.

✔ **Are you involved in any hepatitis C research?** Doctors vary in the amount of time they dedicate to their research and clinical (treating patients) practice.

If you want to determine the doctor's style of management, get the answers to these questions:

✔ **How will you monitor my hep C? How often will I have blood tests?** Regular testing is critical to properly manage your hep C illness.

✔ **Will I need to have a liver biopsy? Are there any alternatives to this procedure?** Liver biopsies are potentially dangerous (see Chapter 7), and practitioners differ in recommendations about their use.

✔ **How do I find out whether your office or the drug companies will work with my insurance company?** Some doctors are more willing to work with you to resolve insurance issues.

Your doctor's answers to the following questions may help you gauge your comfort level with the doctor's approach to drug treatment.

✔ **How many patients do you treat with interferon?** Get a sense of the doctor's experience with combination interferon treatment (see Chapter 8 for more on drug treatment of hep C).

✔ **How do you treat side effects to drug therapy?** You'll want to know whether your doctor is quick to detect drug side effects and remove the drug if it's causing harm.

✔ **Do you feel that the current drug treatment is for me, or should I wait for new treatments?** You'll get an idea of the doctor's treatment style from her answers to this question. Some doctors take an aggressive approach toward current treatment, and others have a more conservative wait-and-see style (see Chapter 8).

✔ **What's your approach with people who don't respond to drug therapy?** Although you hope to be one of the responders, you need to have a plan in place in case you aren't.

✔ **Do you participate in clinical trials for hepatitis C?** This information may be relevant to you if you want to join a clinical trial for a new drug.

You also want to know whether the doctor is open-minded and will work with you or your other healthcare providers in certain situations. Ask these questions to find out:

✔ **Will you help me in using integrative or alternative therapies in addition to or instead of drugs?** Doctors vary in their knowledge about and opinion of complementary and alternative medicine (CAM).

• Your doctor may be extremely knowledgeable about and supportive of CAM, and may actively work with alternative providers for hepatitis C.

• Other doctors may not know very much about CAM but be willing to monitor you while you pursue other treatments alongside conventional treatment.

• Some doctors may see complementary and alternative treatments as hogwash. This type of prejudice is becoming less frequent as doctors realize that the general public is vastly interested in complementary treatments (see Chapter 10 for a discussion of the National Center for Complementary and Alternative Medicine, a branch of the National Institutes of Health).

✔ **Have you worked with other HIV co-infected people before?** If you are co-infected with HIV and hep C, it's crucial that your doctor has such experience or will work with your HIV doctors.

✔ **What is your approach to working with people with depression, anxiety, or psychological problems?** The chronic illness of hepatitis C and drug treatment can add to these emotional problems. You're trying to find out whether the doctor is compassionate.

✔ **How do you feel about patients who use or have used illegal drugs, alcohol, or cigarettes?** The answer will help you decide whether the doctor is very judgmental about personal aspects of your medical history. If you still use any substances, find out whether the doctor will be supportive of your situation.

People with Hep C rank their doctors

A report published in the April 2004 issue of the medical journal *Hepatology* studied one group of people being treated for chronic hepatitis C.

Within this particular group, 41 percent said they had communication problems with their doctor. Of those people:

✔ Twenty-eight percent reported communication problems with their doctors and said the problems were due to feeling rushed, ignored, or not listened to, or being treated poorly.

✔ Twenty-three percent thought their doctors did a poor job in their diagnosis and treatment.

✔ Nine percent felt stigmatized by their doctor as sexually promiscuous or drug addicts.

People who didn't respond to the drug treatment were more likely to have communication problems with their doctor. The researchers who performed the study wondered whether poor communication between doctor and patient turned into poor compliance (not taking all the medication correctly). Patients who don't take their medication correctly may not have a complete response to the medication.

My take on the message for people with hep C is: Get a doctor who treats you with respect, take all your medication, and see your doctor *immediately* if you have any problems with your medication.

You may also want to find out how your doctor deals with folks with advanced chronic hepatitis C disease.

✔ **What happens if I get seriously ill?** Find out which local hospitals your doctor is associated with.

✔ **Have any of your patients had a liver transplant?** Here's your chance to find out your physician's experience with this serious situation. Read more about transplants in Chapter 9.

Find the answer to these questions concerning the logistical aspects of the doctor's office:

✔ **Does the doctor have available appointments for you at the time you need?**

✔ **Is the doctor's office within a reasonable traveling distance?**

✔ **How well does your doctor's office communicate with you about results of your tests?**

You might also speak to other people with hep C to find out about their doctors. But remember that each of you might have different personal responses to the same physician. A certain chemistry exists between the healthcare provider and the client/patient that's completely individual.

Creating Your Hep C Notebook

Keeping all your medical information up-to-date and in one place is a good idea. Your best bet is to assemble some sort of notebook where you can store everything. You can use an actual notebook, a three-ring binder (and a hole puncher), a folder, or any combination of these. Whatever system you use, keep the information organized and easy to find. Include the following types of information:

- **Results of lab tests and other diagnostic procedures:** Include such things as blood test results, scanning results, biopsy reports, and other diagnostic information. Here are some tips on maintaining those records:

  - Request copies of the results of every single test you take. Ask as soon as you have the test or when you first get the result. You may have to pay for copies in some instances.

  - Consider using a ringed notebook. The documents won't fall out, and you can access them easily.

  - Make sure the name of the test, the results, and the test or procedure date are legible.

- **Diary of symptoms:** You can write this on loose-leaf paper to keep in your ringed notebook or in a separate bound notebook with lined paper. Make sure to date each entry, and write down when the symptom started and when it disappeared or was treated. You may have daily entries to record how you feel each day. This information is an essential part of monitoring your treatment.

- **List of prescription and over-the-counter medications, vitamins, and minerals you take:** Go through your medicine cabinet, and write down each one. Include the amount (50 mg, 100 mg, and so on) and how often you take it (once a day, once a week, and so on).

- **List of questions:** Write down questions you have for your doctor and other healthcare professionals and keep the answers when you get them.

  ✔ **List of doctor visits:** For each visit, write down any information or advice the doctor gives you. This information also helps you keep track of health insurance and payment issues.

  ✔ **General information on hepatitis C:** Include material that you receive from doctors, drug companies, the American Liver Foundation, and so on. Depending on how much information you have, you can place this info in your ringed notebook or folders.

  ✔ **Food diary:** Some practitioners ask you to keep a food diary. As you do with the diary of symptoms, you can keep a record of what you're eating so that if you have a problem, you can figure out which foods may have caused it. Read more about nutrition and issues of food and hep C in Chapter 11.

When your first notebook is full, get another, and keep collecting all your information. Keep your old records and notebooks; they have important information you might need at some point.

Get creative, and put in healthy affirmations or happy pictures on the front of your notebook or within the pages. Positive thinking can help you get well faster.

Your doctor will appreciate your effort to manage your disease on your end. Having all this information conveniently on hand allows you and your doctor to make the best use of the time you have together during visits — more time for discussions and questions, and less time spent on, "Uh, let me think . . ." and "Now, where did I put that?"

Including Others in Your Healthcare Support

You and your doctor are the backbone of your support system, but you need others to help you out, too. Get as much support as you need from other healthcare practitioners, friends, and family. And keep everyone connected and informed.

Integrating other healthcare providers

In all likelihood, you'll visit other healthcare providers in addition to your primary care provider and liver specialist. All of your healthcare practitioners are part of your medical support team, which may include the following members:

- ✔ **Mental health professionals:** You may be under the treatment of a psychiatrist, psychologist, or social worker.

- ✔ **Other medical specialists:** You may be undergoing treatment or taking medication for other medical conditions, such as high blood pressure or diabetes.

- ✔ **Complementary and alternative practitioners:** You might visit an acupuncturist, herbalist, naturopathic doctor, massage or reiki therapist, homeopath, or ayurvedic practitioner. I discuss these approaches in Chapters 10 and 13.

 Keep all your practitioners informed about *all* of your healthcare issues. Your medical doctor who treats your hepatitis C, in particular, needs to know about all other medications and treatments. The liver is a sensitive organ, and many herbs and medications have the potential to cause damage (see Chapter 12).

 Refer to your healthcare notebook to exchange information between your practitioners. You can bring copies of test results from one provider and give to another doctor.

Bringing in friends and family

 Friends and family also have a key role to play in your support system. When you're fatigued, depressed, or suffering from other symptoms or side effects of medication, call in your support team! You may need someone to drive you to appointments, pick up medication, or call your doctor. I include a separate chapter in this book — Chapter 19 — just for friends and family who want to know how they can help you.

Bring someone — a friend, family member, or support group person — to your appointments with doctors or alternative healthcare providers to help you remember what the doctor tells you. When your doctor answers your questions, gives you test results, or explains specific details of your condition, you may have trouble remembering everything he said. Fuzzy thinking can be a symptom of hepatitis C, and simply being in a doctor's office can be pretty stressful and make it hard to remember everything. Two heads are better than one when it comes to remembering the important info from your doctor's visit.

 You should write down the important info about each visit while sitting in the doctor's office or immediately afterward.

Chapter 6

Testing for the Hepatitis C Virus

. . . .

In This Chapter

▶ Starting the testing process

▶ Looking at the different types of hepatitis C tests

▶ Understanding the results of your hepatitis C tests

▶ Determining your (geno)type of hepatitis C virus

▶ Keeping track of your tests

. . . .

Many people have absolutely no idea that the hepatitis C virus is swimming around in their blood and lounging in their liver. You may not have symptoms that lead you to a doctor until years or decades after infection. By that time, irreversible damage could occur. The sooner you know you have hep C, the sooner you can take the action described in this book to save your liver and to prevent the spread of hep C to others.

The hep C virus tests tell you whether you've ever been infected and if you're infected now. Whether you're a newbie or a veteran hep C virus test-taker, I give you a handle on interpreting your results.

New and improved tests are being developed all the time. The tests available today are more accurate and have a better ability to detect virus than tests from just a few years ago. Your liver specialist will have the latest information on any new tests.

Beginning the Process

If you're thinking about taking a hepatitis C test or if you've recently taken a test, consider this: Knowledge is power. Determining whether you've been infected and knowing for sure whether the virus is in your blood will either ease your mind or serve as the first step on the hepatitis C recovery journey.

In a nutshell, here's how it works: Hep C tests involve drawing blood, and sometimes, there are lots of them. A white-coated person draws blood from a vein in your arm, and the blood is then transferred into different test tubes with a variety of color-coded tops, to be shipped away for specialty laboratory testing. If you perform the first test yourself (see the section "Places to get tested," later in this chapter), you perform the blood-drawing duties by puncturing your finger with a lancet.

Waiting for test results can be nerve-wracking — especially in the beginning. It can take anywhere from a few days to a couple of weeks to get your results. Use this time to get your support system going and bone up on your health insurance policy (all topics covered in Part III). Try to stay calm while you wait!

The laboratory sends or faxes your results to your healthcare practitioner, who in turn calls you immediately or tells you the results at your scheduled follow-up visit. The more proactive you can be in following up and keeping track of your results, the less anxious you will feel.

Reasons to get tested

The hepatitis C infection is usually silent. It acts like a character in a movie who sneaks around in the shadows while he goes about his dirty tricks.

How do you know whether you should look for hep C in your blood? You may want to get tested if any of these situations apply to you:

- ✔ You've experienced a risky exposure sometime, somewhere. (I cover the topic of hep C transmission in Chapter 2, but I also help you weigh possible exposures later in this section.)
- ✔ You found out you have high liver enzymes during a routine blood test. (I cover liver enzymes in Chapter 7.)
- ✔ You have symptoms such as fatigue or abdominal pain (read about symptoms of hep C in Chapter 4).

With the latter two situations, your doctor is likely on the case already. But with exposure, you may be sorting it out yourself.

Here are some questions to help you decide whether you've had any risky exposures. Like pregnancy, it has to happen only once.

Can you answer yes to any one of these questions?

- ✔ Did you receive clotting-factor concentrates before 1987? (Beginning at that time, clotting factors were treated against human immunodeficiency virus, which also protected against hep C virus.)
- ✔ Have you ever shared needles or other drug paraphernalia?
- ✔ Have you had long-term dialysis?
- ✔ Did you receive a blood transfusion or organ transplant before 1992 (when the hep C test was first used for screening)?
- ✔ Have you had tattoos or body piercing performed with unsanitary, shared instruments (such as in prison)?
- ✔ Have you had a needlestick or puncture accident as a health-care worker?
- ✔ Were you born to a hepatitis C–infected mother?
- ✔ Do you have HIV infection?
- ✔ Were you exposed to blood in a military setting?
- ✔ Are you the spouse or sex partner of someone with hep C?

If you answered yes to *any* of these questions, you may have been exposed to hep C. Check out Chapter 2 for the complete scoop on transmission of the disease.

Places to get tested

The best place to get your first test is your healthcare practitioner's office. Later on, if you find out that you do have hep C, you'll be referred to a liver specialist who's more knowledgeable about the ins and outs of testing.

If you don't have insurance, or you want more confidentiality, you can find a nearby clinic by calling your local health department. Clinics for people with HIV or sexually transmitted diseases, intravenous drug users, or homeless people may also provide hep C testing. These clinics usually provide some sort of counseling and advice so you can follow up any result as wisely as any owl.

Another option is a *home testing kit.* You can buy a screening test kit (which tests for antibodies; see the "Getting Tested" section, later in the chapter) at your local pharmacy, by telephone, or on the Web. To contact Home Access Health Corporation, which makes a hepatitis C test for home use, call its hepatitis C information line: 888-888-HEPC (888-888-4372) or check out its Web site (www.homeaccess.com).

Here's how it works: You collect your blood at home, send it to the laboratory, and then call for the confidential results and counseling about the next step to take. Make sure to follow the detailed instructions exactly to a T, or you may not get an accurate result. Be sure to speak with your doctor if your test results are positive.

Getting Tested

Welcome to the world of high-tech testing. Like other types of medical tests, looking for virus is a matter of medical sleuthing. The goal here is to examine your blood, attempting to detect signs of the hep C virus.

The latest technology is used to test your blood for signs, or *markers,* of hep C infection. The tests are divided into two categories, according to which marker — antibodies or RNA — you're looking for.

All about antibodies

We all have millions of antibodies in our blood. We start making them in childhood. Breastfeeding mothers give antibodies to their babies through milk. At about 6 months, infants start to make their own antibodies. The purpose of vaccination is to get humans to produce antibodies against the vaccine, which looks like the virus or bacteria we want to fight.

When exposed to a virus, bacteria, or even a vaccine, your immune system makes a specific antibody against these agents. The antibody is like a key that fits a "lock," or *antigen* component, of the virus, bacteria, or vaccine. In the best-case scenario, your antibody *neutralizes* or blocks the effect of the foreign antigen.

Unfortunately, like any ammunition, your antibody may fail in one of two ways. It may have no effect. For example, the antibodies that the anti-hep C tests detect aren't neutralizing antibodies. Or, worse, the antibody can backfire and hurt you. For example, autoimmune diseases like lupus are caused by antibodies that attack the body. Some people with hepatitis C develop autoimmune diseases, and medical researchers are trying to discover the interaction of hepatitis C and autoimmunity.

Analyzing your antibodies

Antibody testing answers one question: Have I been infected? The antibody test does *not* tell if you are currently infected. It says only whether you've been infected at some point of your life.

Your immune response makes *antibodies* after you're infected by hepatitis C. The human body makes millions of different types of antibodies to fight millions of different types of invaders — of which hepatitis C is only one. Antibodies usually show up a few months after the initial infection. (For more on antibodies, see the "All about antibodies" sidebar in this chapter. And for more on the immune response to hepatitis C virus, see Chapter 3.)

Meeting the tests

Antibody tests look for the antibody to hep C (which answers to the name *anti-hep C* or *anti-HCV*). The presence of these antibodies tells you and your doctor that you've been infected with hep C at some point in your life. In the testing world, these are the first tests performed, because they're the quickest and cheapest. Antibody tests come in a few varieties:

- ✔ **EIA (enzyme immunoassay):** This test can also be called ELISA. Newer generations of these tests are quite accurate, with fewer false negative or positive results than earlier versions.

- ✔ **RIBA (recombinant immunoblot assay):** This test is sometimes used as a second antibody test. It was more commonly used with earlier-generation EIA tests.

The names of these tests — and the RNA tests that I cover in the aptly named "Reading your RNA results" section, later in the chapter — are about the complex technical detective systems, rather than the function of the test itself.

Reading the results

The waiting is over. You have results in hand, and you want to know more. Here are some ways to interpret your results (and check out Table 6-1 for an easily accessible summary):

- ✔ **Nonreactive (without symptoms or history of exposure):** Congratulations! You're free and clear! No further testing is needed. Don't forget to protect yourself from future exposure to the hep C virus (see Chapter 2 to read about transmission).

- ✔ **Nonreactive (with symptoms or history of exposure):** Your doctor will perform further testing — either an RNA test or a retest of your antibody levels after a few months — to see which of these categories you fit into:

- You don't have hep C infection. You may have another liver disease.

- You're infected with hep C but haven't made antibodies because it's too soon after infection (it can take a few months to make antibodies).

- You may have hepatitis C, but you're just one of those rare people who don't make the antibodies to hep C.

✔ **Reactive:** This result means that you have anti-hep C antibodies in your blood. Your doctor will follow up this result with:

- A viral RNA test (see the next section) to see if you have virus in your blood

- Liver blood tests (see Chapter 7) to see if you have any damage to your liver

Table 6-1		**Hep C Antibody Tests and Results**	
Purpose of Test	**Test Name(s)**	**Possible Results**	**Normal Range***
Hep C Virus Antibody Screening/Detection	EIA ELISA	Reactive Indeterminate Nonreactive	Nonreactive
Hep C Virus Antibody Confirmation	RIBA	Reactive Indeterminate Nonreactive	Nonreactive

* Normal range is listed on the laboratory report as the result for a healthy uninfected person.

You may be one of the many folks who go to give blood and find out you test positive for hepatitis C! After you get over your initial shock, call your primary care physician, and schedule an appointment to follow up this result. You may find that you were infected in the past but that you're no longer infected, or you may find that you have hepatitis C right now and didn't know it. If you currently have hep C, it's actually a good thing that you found out about it early — you can now get yourself under the care of a good liver specialist (see Chapter 5) and start focusing on healthy living (see Part III).

In the past, screening tests by blood banks for hepatitis C sometimes yielded false positive results. Steps were taken to reduce the number of false positive results, but it's always possible that your positive result was an error. The only way to know for sure is to see your doctor and get follow-up tests (see the "Regarding your hepatitis C RNA" section, later in the chapter).

Antibodies for life?

Like a good vaccine that immunizes long term after just one shot, your hep C antibodies may stay around for years. So even if you have successful treatment for hepatitis C, and your virus is gone, the antibody test (but not the RNA test) may stay positive. Be prepared for this situation if your blood is tested for job or insurance purposes. (I discuss finances and the workplace in Chapter 16.)

Don't panic. Some researchers report that the antibodies will eventually disappear — after the hep C is gone. Research is under way to find out how long antibodies last after the hep C virus is gone.

Regarding your hepatitis C RNA

Hep C RNA tests detect virus in your bloodstream. Your doctor will order these lab tests for you during your care for hepatitis C:

✔ When you first test positive during an antibody test

✔ Before, during, and after treatment with combination peginterferon (see Chapter 8)

✔ During your continuing care for hepatitis C

RNA is the abbreviation for *ribonucleic acid*. RNA is almost an exact mirror image of the better-known DNA *(deoxyribonucleic acid)*. Our genes come in the form of DNA, and hep C genes come in the form of RNA. (See Chapter 3 to read more about DNA and RNA.)

Meeting the tests

RNA tests are used to detect the presence of a virus. Have you seen a cop show in which the detective tests crime-scene blood for a suspect's DNA? Here, hepatitis C is the prime suspect. Finding hep C RNA in your blood means that you have a current infection.

You may wonder why tests look for RNA and not the virus itself. Remember that the hep C virus is minuscule and can't even be seen with a regular microscope. RNA, being a nucleic acid, can be detected in very small amounts by certain high-tech biological tests (similar to the ones done in forensic science). The purpose of detection here is to find evidence of the hepatitis C virus.

There are two types of RNA tests. The *qualitative RNA test* gives a yes or no answer — yes, you have the virus, or no, you don't. The *quantitative RNA test* estimates the levels of hep C RNA in your blood — which is called your *viral load.* While the two types of RNA tests really answer the same question about whether you're currently infected with the hepatitis C virus, the quantitative test goes a step further by giving an idea of how much virus you have.

Qualitative tests use PCR- (polymerase chain reaction) and TMA- (transcription mediated assay) based technologies to detect hep C RNA. Viral load (quantitative) tests use PCR and TMA technologies, in addition to bDNA (branched DNA) technologies.

Your liver doctor will choose the test that's most appropriate for you out of the many that are now offered. For example, one major U.S. laboratory testing company, Quest Diagnostics, offers three different qualitative hep C RNA tests and six different quantitative hep C RNA tests.

Quest Diagnostics has lots of information on hepatitis C (and other tests) on its Web site (www.questdiagnostics.com) for both consumers and medical professionals.

Some of the newer RNA tests aren't yet FDA approved, even though they may be commonly used, safe, and accurate. This fact can affect an insurance company's decision about coverage. Discuss this situation with your doctor, and see Chapter 16.

Reading the results

Your test results for the qualitative RNA test will come back as positive or negative (which is the same as saying "below the lower level detected by the test"). Results for the quantitative, or viral load, tests are dependent on which test you take (see Table 6-2 for a summary of different test results).

Ask your doctor if she considers your result to be high or low on a quantitative RNA/viral load test. Because each test is different, it's difficult for me to assign high or low values here.

When considering viral load tests, be careful when interpreting your numbers:

- ✔ Different tests come up with slightly different results. Tests from different manufacturers have the same overall interpretation, but the exact number differs because of slightly different techniques.

> ✔ Also, your exact number varies from day to day. Don't get too queasy about this, but remember that the virus is alive and growing and dying each day. So each test is like a separate snapshot of how much virus is in your blood.

Your viral load is important because lower viral loads may be easier to treat with peginterferon medication (see Chapter 8). During treatment, your doctor will look for changes in your viral load that are 10-fold higher or lower. Going from one million to one hundred thousand is a 10-fold change (1 log); going from one million to ten thousand is a 100-fold change (2 log); and going from one million to one thousand is a 1,000-fold change (3 log).

Table 6-2	Hep C RNA Tests and Results		
Purpose of Test	**Test Name(s)**	**Possible Results**	**Normal Range***
Qualitative Hep C Virus RNA	PCR TMA	Positive Undetectable	Undetectable (Below lower limit of detection of test)
Quantitative Hep C Virus RNA	PCR bDNA TMA	5–50,000,000 IU/ml** (Each test has different lower and upper limits) Undetectable	Undetectable (Below lower limit of detection of test)

*Normal range is listed on the laboratory report as the result for a healthy uninfected person.

**Previous tests give results as copies of RNA. In general, each IU is about one to five copies of RNA, depending on the type of test.

Be responsible. If you have a positive result on *any* viral RNA test, you are potentially infectious to others. Take precautions to keep others safe (for more information, see Chapter 2).

Even if you test positive for hep C RNA, you may not have any symptoms of hepatitis C. You might remain forever asymptomatic (without symptoms) or develop them in the years to come. The value of getting tested is to find out about your hepatitis C before serious symptoms occur so you can take action by getting proper medical treatment.

You may have an RNA test to see if your combination peginterferon is reducing your viral load. If you still have the virus, your doctor can help you determine what other treatments may be available to you now or down the road. Don't forget to do your own work to stay healthy by eating your vegetables, avoiding toxins, exercising, reducing stress, keeping a positive outlook, and following the other nifty suggestions in Part III.

Genotyping Your Virus

All hep C viruses aren't exactly alike, according to scientists who looked at hep C from all over the world. It turns out that the hep C critters have some differences in their genetic structure. Hep C is classified into at least six distinct types called *genotypes*. The genotypes have been further divided into more than 50 subtypes, which have a letter after their name — genotype 1a and genotype 1b are subtypes of genotype 1, for example.

It's possible to have any genotype no matter where you become infected, but some genotypes are more common in certain parts of the world.

- ✔ Genotype 1 is the most common genotype in North and South America, Europe, Australia, and Japan.
- ✔ Genotypes 2 and 3 are the next most common subtypes in North and South America, Europe, Australia, and Japan.
- ✔ Genotype 4 is the most common genotype in the Middle East and Africa.
- ✔ Genotype 5 is the most common genotype in South Africa.
- ✔ Genotype 6 is the most common genotype in Southeast Asia.

A genotyping test, which is performed after you've already had a positive hep C RNA test, uses the hep C RNA to classify the type of hep C virus you have. You need to have this test only once, because your genotype stays the same (unless you're exposed to hepatitis C again).

The reason your doctor will test your blood to determine your hep C genotype is that it might be important when considering combination peginterferon. Your genotype is *one* factor that determines how well and how quickly interferon combination therapy (see Chapter 8) will rid you of hep C. Genotypes 2 and 3 respond the best and quickest. But don't despair if you're not genotype 2 or 3! Knowing your genotype will help your doctor plan the treatment strategy that works best for you.

A hot area of research focuses on finding anything else the genotype differences might predict. An ongoing debate concerns whether certain hep C genotypes cause more severe disease. So far, the studies are not conclusive. For now, the main reasons to test genotype is to plan drug treatment.

Charting Your Progress

As you can see by reading this chapter, hep C is often all about tests, tests, and more tests. Try to get copies of any of your tests, and if you're thinking about starting a healthcare notebook to keep all your hep C stuff together (as I discuss in Chapter 5), file them there.

But even if you have copies of the results, the sheer amount of paperwork can quickly build up. So you may find it helpful to simplify your records by creating a chart on which you write down the names, dates, and results of your tests, along with any burning questions you may have about them for your doctor. Creating a chart can also help you track the progression of your test results at a glance. To make things easy, you can just photocopy Figure 6-1 and stick it in your notebook (or fill it out right here).

TEST RESULTS

Date	Test/Result	Question(s)	Answer(s)

Figure 6-1: Photocopy this page to include in your Hep C notebook.

Chapter 7

Testing the Liver

● ●

In This Chapter

▶ Analyzing your blood for liver enzymes and function

▶ Scanning your liver

▶ Getting a liver biopsy

● ●

You know you've been infected with hepatitis C (see Chapter 6). Now your liver doctor wants to perform laboratory tests to predict the condition of your liver.

Blood tests for substances made by the liver can detect evidence of liver damage. Your doctor will also order an ultrasound of your liver or maybe a CT or MRI scan. The riskiest test, but also the most informative, is the liver biopsy, which involves the removal of a tiny piece of your liver that's then analyzed under a microscope.

In this chapter, I describe the different types of tests, any risks involved, and how to interpret your results. Your doctor will use the information he gets from these liver tests, along with results from your hepatitis C virus tests (see Chapter 6), and what you tell him about your symptoms to diagnose and treat you.

 Just because you've had a past or even a current hepatitis C infection doesn't mean you have liver disease. Some people have no symptoms or signs of liver disease. Your doctor will take tests regularly to keep on top of any liver problems that may occur.

Blood Tests

When you go for a physical, your healthcare practitioner frequently orders blood tests. Many folks first find out they have hep C after undergoing a routine blood test and finding that one or more of the tests is abnormal. In this section, I outline tests your doctor may order to define the nature of your liver damage, including some of which are included in the tests you undergo during a physical.

By using results from different tests, your doctor can perform a differential diagnosis and rule out other non-hepatitis C–related diseases or differentiate between different stages of hepatitis C disease.

After your blood is drawn, it's sent to a medical laboratory, where technicians use computerized machines to perform tests. The results from your tests are compared to reference ranges. A *reference range* is a group of numbers — from low to high — that includes the results of 95 percent of healthy people (5 percent of healthy people will have results outside of the reference range). The reference range used to be called a *normal range*. What's normal or average for one group of people of a certain age or gender will differ from that of another group of people. Different laboratories themselves have different reference ranges. If your test result is higher or lower than the reference range, the number is flagged with an L or H (for low or high).

Inform your doctor of any medications you're taking because they can affect your test results. Other factors that can affect your test results include:

✔ Your gender

✔ Your age

✔ Whether you're fasting at the time of the test

✔ Strenuous exercise

✔ Alcohol and drug use

Obtain and keep copies of your laboratory test results (see Chapter 5 for advice on managing your personal hep C medical information). The name of the laboratory, your name, the test date, and your doctor's name appear on the test results.

It's up to your healthcare provider to interpret your results. The lab may flag small differences in your results from the reference range, but your doctor may not feel that the difference is big enough to be of concern. Your doctor may want to repeat your test if one number is extremely high or low, or wait a few months and test you again.

In the following sections, I list some blood tests that are commonly used to diagnose liver disease; your practitioner will use some of these, as well as other tests, to study your individual situation.

Liver enzyme and liver function tests

There's no one test that indicates chronic hepatitis C disease.
Tests for the effects of hepatitis C on your liver include:

✔ **Liver enzyme tests:** These tests measure current liver cell
injury by the amount of enzymes that are "leaked" out of damaged or dying liver cells. (See Chapter 3 for more information
on enzymes.)

✔ **Liver function tests:** These tests look at levels of proteins
made by the liver. If your liver damage is such that your liver
function is impaired, levels of these proteins will be low. If
your bilirubin, clotting factors, or albumin levels are low, you
may have cirrhosis or late-stage liver disease.

In the following sections, I discuss some of the tests that fall into
these categories. Check out Table 7-1 for a quick summary and a
list of sample reference ranges for each test covered.

Table 7-1	Liver Blood Tests at a Glance
Liver Enzyme Tests	*Sample Reference Ranges**
ALT	0–35 u/ml
AST	17–59 IU/L
ALP	44–147 IU/L
GGT	0–51 IU/L
5'N'Tase	2–17 U/L
Albumin	3.5–5.5 g/dl
Bilirubin (total)	0.3–1.9 mg/dl
Prothrombin time	11.0–13.5 seconds

** The numbers given here are sample average reference ranges. Your laboratory will have
different reference ranges. And your results can be adequately interpreted only by your
healthcare professional.*
*Note: Abbreviations used in this table: u = units; ml = milliliter; IU = International Units; L = liter;
g = gram; dl = deciliter; mg = milligrams.*

ALT

Small amounts of ALT (alanine aminotransferase) are normally found in blood. When the liver is damaged, ALT is released into the bloodstream. ALT is found in organs other than the liver (kidneys, heart, muscles, and pancreas), but most increases in ALT are from liver damage.

ALT processes the amino acid alanine, which is one of the 20 amino acid protein building blocks. ALT is also called SGPT (serum glutamate pyruvate transaminase) or alanine transaminase.

AST

AST (aspartate aminotransferase) is also called SGOT (serum glutamic-oxaloacetic transaminase). Like ALT, AST is found mainly in the liver but also in other parts of the body. AST and ALT are usually measured together and are good indicators of liver disease or damage. Sometimes, test results give AST/ALT ratios.

ALP

ALP (alkaline phosphatase) is found in all parts of the body, with particularly high concentrations in the liver, bone, and placenta (during pregnancy). Like ALT and AST, ALP might leak into the bloodstream when liver cells are damaged as a result of hepatitis C. Children (who have growing bones), pregnant women (especially in their last trimester), and people with bone disease also have higher levels of ALP.

GGT

GGT refers to gamma-glutamyl transferase, but it's also called gamma-glutamyl transpeptidase (GGTP) or Gamma-GT. High levels of GGT are found in the liver, bile ducts, and the kidney. Bloodstream GGT levels will be higher in people with diseases of the liver and bile ducts.

5'N'Tase

Higher levels of the enzyme 5'N'Tase (5'nucleotidase), also known as 5'NT, in your blood indicate a problem with bile secretion. Hepatitis or cirrhosis can cause a blockage of bile flow.

Albumin

Albumin is the major blood protein made by the liver. One function of albumin is to keep the blood from leaking through the blood vessels, which can cause fluid retention in the ankles (*edema*), lungs, or abdomen (*ascites*). Low levels of albumin may be due to liver or kidney disease, malnutrition, or even a low-protein diet.

Bilirubin

This pigmented (yellow) waste chemical comes from the normal process of red blood cells' dying after 90 to 120 days. A healthy liver converts bilirubin and sends it out of the body with the bile that goes to the intestine. Excreted bilirubin gives feces (stools) their characteristic brownish color.

When the liver is diseased, bilirubin isn't converted and excreted. Stools might, therefore, be light-colored. The bilirubin that's not properly excreted builds up in the body and gives a yellowish color to skin and eyes (a condition known as *jaundice*) and dark brown tea color to urine.

High levels of bilirubin are due to either too much production of bilirubin (from red blood cells dying) or because the liver isn't processing bilirubin, which happens when the liver is damaged. This is one of three tests used to determine wait time for a liver transplant (see Chapter 9).

In addition to using a blood test, urine can be tested for bilirubin.

PT test

The PT (prothrombin time) test measures how quickly your blood clots, which is dependent on clotting factors (proteins) that are made by the liver. The PT test is used as a marker of advanced liver disease and can indicate blood-clotting problems where it takes you longer to stop bleeding.

Your laboratory may also give PT results that have been converted to an internationally recognized and easily comparable value that's called the International Normalized Ratio (INR). The INR is one of the three factors used to determine wait time for a liver transplant.

Other blood tests

Additional tests that measure other markers in your blood give your doctor a clearer picture of any liver disease and also any effects from the combination peginterferon drug treatment (see Chapter 8).

Complete blood count (CBC)

A complete blood count (CBC) looks at the number and types of cells in your blood. Your doctor will look for problems such as

✔ **Reduced white blood cells or platelets:** This may indicate portal hypertension, a complication of cirrhosis in which pressures are increased in the portal vein. (see Chapter 4).

✔ **Indicators of anemia:** This problem is very common during ribivarin treatment.

The complete blood count includes the following tests:

✔ **White blood cell (WBC) count:** The total number of white blood cells. Changes can indicate problems of hepatitis C infection or side effects of interferon treatment. Interferon can cause *neutropenia,* which is a decrease in *neutrophils,* one type of white blood cell.

✔ **Red blood cell (RBC) count:** The total number of red blood cells. Low levels can indicate anemia.

✔ **Hematocrit (HCT):** Percentage of blood cells that are red blood cells. Low levels can indicate anemia.

✔ **Hemoglobin:** The amount of this oxygen-carrying protein. Low levels can indicate anemia.

✔ **Platelet count:** Number of platelets in your blood (may be altered in cirrhosis).

AFP

Tests for AFP (alpha-fetoprotein) are used to screen for liver cancer in people with cirrhosis. But not everyone with liver cancer has this marker. Pregnant women usually have higher levels of this protein, which is also used to look for problems in pregnancy. You may have slightly high levels of this protein if you have hepatitis or cirrhosis.

Iron

The liver stores iron, and an overabundance of iron (iron overload) can add to the damage caused by hepatitis C. Too much iron can be a problem during interferon treatment (see Chapter 8). See your physician to determine whether you should avoid supplements that include iron.

Creatinine

Creatinine is actually a breakdown product of creatine, which is made by the liver and transported to your muscles. The kidneys excrete the waste product creatinine, and when your kidneys are damaged, creatinine levels rise. When the liver stops functioning in end-stage liver disease, this can cause serious kidney problems as well. This test is one of the three used to determine your wait time for a liver transplant (see Chapter 9).

Imaging Tests

Images from ultrasounds, CT (or CAT) scans, and MRIs give a picture of the overall size and shape of your liver. You'll probably get an initial ultrasound when you're first diagnosed with hepatitis C. If you have cirrhosis, you'll have ultrasounds once or twice a year to screen for liver cancer. CT scans and MRIs are used to further visualize liver tumors.

Imaging studies, particularly MRI and CAT scans, are expensive. Make sure you're covered by your insurance.

Scanning tests allow your doctor to get an image of your liver from the outside of your body. Because these tests are noninvasive, you have less chance of any side effects than with a liver biopsy.

If you have an implantable cardiac defibrillator or pacemaker, you can't have an MRI test. If you're pregnant, you can't have a CAT scan, and ultrasound is more widely used in pregnancy than an MRI.

Ultrasound

Ultrasound uses sound waves to produce an image of your liver. No X-rays or other types of radiation are used. A technician places a gel on your skin to help transmit the sound waves and rubs a small wand over your abdominal area to get a picture on the computer screen. You may have to move to one side of your body or another to enable the technician to get a complete picture of your liver.

CT or CAT scan

A CT (computed tomography) scan, also called a CAT (computerized axial tomography) scan, is a special type of X-ray that scans an area of the body in layers (slices) that are analyzed by a computer. When doctors are looking for the possibility of cirrhosis or liver cancer, they use CT scans as a follow-up when ultrasound results are unclear.

MRI

MRI (magnetic resonance imaging) scans use radio waves and strong magnets rather than X-rays. A computer analyzes the signals from the MRI to give detailed information about your liver. MRI scans are helpful to look at liver cancers and can sometimes tell a benign tumor from a cancerous one. In MRI scans, which take longer than CT scans, patients are in an enclosed tubelike machine.

Liver Biopsy

After you're first diagnosed with hepatitis C, your doctor will want to see how much damage there is to your liver. Though liver enzyme and liver function blood tests give valuable information, a liver biopsy is currently considered the gold standard for noting any inflammation or fibrosis damage caused by hepatitis C. Your doctor will use a thin needle to remove a tiny piece of your liver, which will be examined under a microscope.

The most commonly performed type of biopsy is a *percutaneous biopsy,* which is what I describe in this section. Other types of liver biopsies are sometimes used if you have symptoms (such as a bleeding disorder) that would make this type of biopsy dangerous.

Talking about timing

Doctors differ in how often they prescribe biopsies. Many doctors perform a biopsy when you first find out about your hep C. The information from the biopsy is used as a baseline to see how serious your hep C disease is.

A main purpose of the biopsy is help in decisions about drug treatment. Some doctors don't perform biopsies on people with genotypes 2 or 3 (see Chapter 6). Because these genotypes respond well to combination peginterferon treatment (see Chapter 8), your doctor may suggest treatment in the absence of a biopsy. For people with genotype 1, for whom treatment works about half the time, your doctor may want to perform a biopsy to see the status of your liver disease before making a recommendation about treatment.

A biopsy isn't recommended for people with advanced liver disease because the complications of the biopsy could worsen their situation. For people with these diagnoses, direct liver tests (bilirubin, albumin, and prothrombin time, as discussed earlier in this chapter) can provide the necessary information on the progress of their liver disease.

After you've been successfully treated for hep C and no longer have the hep C virus, you no longer need to undergo a biopsy.

Weighing the pros and cons

Only you and your doctor can decide if and when you should have a liver biopsy. Although the liver biopsy provides useful information, consider the risks before agreeing to have one.

The pros

You may feel some relief after having a biopsy because then you know exactly what's going on with your liver. When you're no longer guessing about what damage you have, you can make the best choices to treat your hep C.

Some people who repeatedly have normal ALT and AST liver enzyme levels discover from a biopsy that their liver is scarred with fibrosis. Though this result isn't usual, it does prove that a liver biopsy gives a more definite view of the amount of damage you have sustained from the hep C virus.

The value of a biopsy is to indicate the level of fibrosis so that you can plan a treatment strategy for your hep C. The presence of fibrosis is a marker of possible progression toward cirrhosis (see Chapter 4 for more on the progression). If you have more fibrosis, you may want to take a more aggressive approach. If you have less fibrosis, you may want to take a wait-and-see approach (see the "Interpreting your biopsy results" section, later in the chapter). Either way, the biopsy will give you valuable information.

The cons

The liver biopsy is an invasive procedure, meaning that the biopsy needle goes through your skin and pierces your liver. A small but real risk exists for complications, which occur in about 1 percent of biopsies, or 1 out of 100. A liver biopsy has the following risks:

- ✔ Bleeding that may require blood transfusions or surgery to correct
- ✔ Accidental needle puncture of the lung, intestines, gallbladder, or kidney
- ✔ Abdominal infection
- ✔ Pain

The risk of death from the biopsy is less than 1 in 1,000.

Though usually accurate, a biopsy isn't foolproof in its diagnostic value. For example, the piece of liver taken during your biopsy may not be representative of the disease in your entire liver. Discuss this possibility with your doctor.

Noninvasive alternatives to biopsy are under development; see the section "Evaluating alternatives to biopsy," later in this chapter.

Preparing for your biopsy

Before you can have a biopsy, your doctor will check that you don't have ascites (a complication of cirrhosis) or a bleeding disorder. You may be advised not to take blood thinners — including coumadin, aspirin, ibuprofen, naproxen, vitamin E, and the herb ginkgo biloba —for one week before or after your biopsy.

Before the procedure, you must sign a consent form, fast for six to eight hours, and empty your bladder.

Describing the day of the biopsy

A liver biopsy is usually performed in the outpatient area of a hospital. A hepatologist, gastroenterologist (see Chapter 5 for more on these specialists), or an interventional radiologist performs the biopsy. An *interventional radiologist* is an MD who specializes in minimally invasive surgical procedures that are guided by imaging procedures such as ultrasound, CAT scan, or MRI (see the "Imaging Tests" section, earlier in this chapter). Your doctor might use ultrasound to check placement of the biopsy needle so that he doesn't accidentally puncture another organ.

You may be offered light sedation before the biopsy; this is up to your doctor. You lie down but are awake during the procedure so that you can tell the doctors if you feel severe pain (which is unlikely but could signify a complication). A local anesthetic, similar to that given by a dentist, will numb the biopsy area, which is wiped down with alcohol. You'll be asked to be completely still while a hollow needle is inserted and pulled out, along with a small piece of your liver. The entire procedure takes only a few seconds. You may feel some pain from the needle insertion and removal, like the pain of having your blood drawn.

Afterward, you'll be bandaged up and rolled over onto your right side or asked to remain flat on your back while you stay at the hospital for a few hours so that the staff can monitor you for any complications. Your blood pressure and pulse will be checked regularly. You're asked to stay still to decrease the risk of bleeding. Because the liver has lots of blood vessels, bleeding is the No. 1 risk after a biopsy.

Bring a portable CD player so that you can listen to music or meditations to help you relax while you're in the hospital. Or bring a good book.

As long as you have no complications, you can go home within six hours. For your postbiopsy care, arrange to have someone drive you home because of the sedation, and follow your doctor's advice on follow-up care, rest, and pain relief. You can't use aspirin and ibuprofen, because they can increase bleeding.

Interpreting your biopsy results

A *pathologist* (an MD who specializes in the interpretation of tissue samples) analyzes the sample of your liver and provides your doctor with these results. Your doctor will phone you with biopsy results within a few days or at your next scheduled appointment.

Inflammation and fibrosis are separately measured and graded from 0 to 4 (though other grading systems may have a range from 0 to 6). The higher the number, the greater the amount of inflammation or fibrosis (see Table 7-2). *Fibrosis* is the technical term for scarring of the liver. Extensive fibrosis can lead to cirrhosis, which can develop into end-stage liver disease (see Chapter 4 for more on different forms of disease associated with hepatitis C).

Your biopsy report may also indicate the presence of other problems that might contribute to the disease load on your liver. Deposits of iron could indicate the disease *hemochromatosis* (iron-overload disease), and fat deposits could indicate fatty disease of the liver (nonalcoholic or alcoholic). Your doctor will take these conditions into account when treating your liver disease.

Table 7-2	Scoring Systems for Liver Biopsies	
Grade	*Inflammation*	*Fibrosis*
0	None	None
1	Minimal	Portal fibrosis
2	Mild	Periportal fibrosis
3	Moderate	Bridging fibrosis
4	Severe	Cirrhosis

Based on the info provided by your biopsy, you and your doctor can decide how to proceed with your treatment:

> ✔ Some people with little or no fibrosis decide to take the wait-and-see approach. They may continue eating well (see Chapter 11) and avoiding toxins (see Chapter 12) and wait for

better medications to be available. Chronic hepatitis C may not cause further damage in these people for decades, if ever. Your doctor will order follow-up blood tests to make sure that your disease hasn't progressed, and some doctors perform another biopsy three to five years later.

✔ When your fibrosis is more advanced, or if you have cirrhosis, you may choose to take a more aggressive approach to your treatment and try drug therapy (see Chapter 8), if you haven't already done so.

Evaluating alternatives to biopsy

Noninvasive alternatives are needed to avoid the dangerous side effects that can occur with a liver biopsy. Research is ongoing to find biochemical markers of liver disease that can replace a biopsy.

With late-stage cirrhosis, there's an alternative to liver biopsy: Your doctor can use the results from the tests listed in the "Blood Tests" section, earlier in the chapter, especially liver function and platelet count tests, along with a physical evaluation.

However, for early stages of fibrosis (scarring) and cirrhosis, no set of tests is currently considered to be as accurate as the liver biopsy. The following tests are currently available but are considered *experimental* and may not be covered by your insurance company. You or your doctor may want to consider these tests if the risks of a biopsy are unacceptable:

✔ **FIBROspect II:** This blood test (from Prometheus Laboratories) measures chemicals in the blood and performs a statistical analysis to predict levels of fibrosis.

✔ **Fibrotest and Actitest:** A French company (BioPredictive) has developed these noninvasive panels of tests for fibrosis, which is called the HCV-FibroSure Test in the United States (LabCorp).

Some doctors are using alternative tests in certain people. Future versions of these or other tests may replace at least some of the regular use of liver biopsies for people with hep C.

Chapter 8

Prescribing Medical Treatment

*O*ver the past decade, improvements have been made in conventional medicine for hepatitis C, and research continues to be geared toward treatment with better effectiveness and safety. The primary aim of hepatitis C drug treatment is to protect you from developing cirrhosis, liver failure, or liver cancer. Another level of medical treatment involves those agents that help you cope with symptoms.

In this chapter, I focus on the current best treatment for hep C — combination peginterferon and ribavirin therapy, which works to eliminate hepatitis C virus. I describe what the treatment is all about, who gets treated, and what the side effects and rates of success are. I also touch on treatments for symptoms of chronic hepatitis C, cirrhosis, and liver cancer, as well as medical treatments that are currently in clinical trials.

Here, you can find the information to help you work with your doctor to make the best decisions about treatment.

Describing Interferon Treatment

Variations on interferon treatment have been the mainstay of hepatitis C treatment for many years (see the "Tracing the history of interferon treatment" sidebar in this chapter). At first, interferon was given alone as a *monotherapy*. Now, a form of interferon called peginterferon is used in *combination therapy* with another antiviral drug called ribavirin. The two drugs work much better than either one alone, if you can tolerate the side effects of both drugs.

Defining interferon

Interferon is the name of a type of *cytokine,* which is a protein naturally produced by cells of the body. Interferons fight viral infection; the body makes three classes of interferons, called alpha, beta, and gamma. Drug companies have synthesized a type of the body's alpha interferon and called it *interferon-alfa.*

The different forms of interferon alfa used to treat hepatitis C are:

- ✔ **Interferon alfa 2a and interferon alfa 2b:** These forms are rarely used nowadays, because the more effective pegylated forms are available.

- ✔ **Peginterferon alfa 2a and peginterferon alfa 2b:** These forms are the mainstay of current drug treatment (along with ribavirin, which I describe in the following section).

- ✔ **Consensus interferon:** Another form of interferon alfa, also called *interferon alfacon-1,* which is used when treatment with interferon alfa or peginterferon has failed (see the "Looking at options for nonresponders or relapsers" section, later in the chapter).

Table 8-1 lists these drugs and the manufacturers that produce them.

Peg is an abbreviation for the chemical *polyethylene glycol. Pegylated interferon* is interferon with an added polyethylene glycol molecule. On its own, polyethylene glycol has no noticeable effect on hep C, but when it's attached to interferon, the interferon stays active in the body for a longer period of time. As a result, you can then inject yourself with pegylated interferon, known as *peginterferon,* once a week rather than the three times a week that was necessary with unpegylated interferon. Because peginterferon stays in the body and is easier to use, it gives better results than unpegylated interferon without increasing side effects.

Table 8-1 Antiviral Drugs Used for Hepatitis C Treatment

Drug	Drug Company
Interferon* alfa	
Roferon-A (interferon alfa-2a)	Hoffmann-La Roche
Intron-A (interferon alfa-2b)	Schering-Plough
Peginterferon* alfa	
Pegasys (peginterferon alfa-2a)	Hoffmann-La Roche
Peg-Intron (peginterferon alfa-2b)	Schering-Plough
Consensus Interferon*	
Infergen (interferon alfacon-1)	InterMune
Ribavirin*	
Copegus	Hoffmann-La Roche
Rebetol	Schering-Plough

*Drugs are listed in each category according to their trade name.

Defining ribavirin

Ribavirin is a type of antiviral drug called a *nucleoside analogue.*
(*Nucleosides* are the chemicals that make up DNA and RNA.) With
hepatitis C, ribavirin has no effect on its own. The combination of
interferon alfa or peginterferon alfa plus ribavirin gives greater
effectiveness against hepatitis C virus than either type of interferon
alfa alone. Ribavirin is given in tablet form and is taken orally, with
the amount varying depending on your weight. (Ribavirin is used
in an aerosol form to treat other viral diseases.)

Although combining ribavirin with interferon alfa increases the
antiviral effect, it also increases the number of potential side effects.
Ribavirin is responsible for causing anemia and is extremely dangerous to take while pregnant.

Taking peginterferon plus ribavirin

If your doctor prescribes antiviral medicines for you, you'll inject
the peginterferon weekly and take the ribavirin in pill form daily.
Both drug companies that produce the peginterferon treatment
have come up with easier ways to give yourself an injection: pre-
filled syringes and injection "pens."

Tracing the history of interferon therapy

Interferon was used as a treatment for hep C before the virus was even named — back when it still called hepatitis non-A non-B! Here's a brief look at how we got to where we're at:

✔ In 1986, six months of interferon gave a *sustained virologic response* (SVR) — meaning that at the end of treatment and six months after that, the individual had no hep C virus in his or her blood — in 6 percent of people treated.

✔ The duration of interferon treatment times increased, and so did the response rates.

✔ Ribavirin was added to the therapy and approved by the Food and Drug Administration (FDA) in 1998. Twelve months of interferon plus ribavirin gave a 42 percent SVR rate.

✔ In 2001, pegylated (peg) interferon was used alone.

✔ In 2002, a combination treatment of peginterferon and ribavirin was used. By 2004, changes in length of treatment have led to response rates as high as 80 percent for people with genotype 2 and 50 percent for genotype 1.

✔ In 2005 and beyond, expect different forms of interferon and ribavirin as well as new forms of antiviral medications (not based on interferon or ribavirin), with fewer side effects and improved ability to kill virus in more people with hepatitis C.

Peginterferon plus ribavirin therapy typically lasts 24 to 48 weeks You'll have to visit the doctor weekly for blood tests in the beginning of treatment and then monthly for the remainder of your treatment. Your doctor's office will set up a schedule for you.

Follow the directions that come with the medication exactly and ask your doctor if you have any questions. Use a different injection site each time and dispose of the syringe in a container designed specifically for sharps.

Deciding Whether You're a Prime Candidate

The hepatitis C treatment process isn't easy, and it isn't for everyone. Because of the possibility of serious side effects with peginterferon and ribavirin, undergoing treatment isn't a decision to take lightly.

Your doctor will carefully evaluate the type and progression of your disease, your overall health, factors that may rule out treatment, your commitment to seeing the process through, and whether the timing is appropriate. After these evaluations, your doctor will give you his opinion on whether peginterferon plus ribavirin therapy will have enough potential benefit. Because of the serious side effects of peginterferon plus ribavirin (see the "Understanding the Side Effects" section, later in the chapter), it's important to determine whether you

✔ Should get treated because you're at a high risk for developing cirrhosis. Your liver biopsy would show evidence of fibrosis, which is the precursor of cirrhosis. Or perhaps you have cirrhosis already, and you want to prevent development of decompensated cirrhosis.

✔ Shouldn't take the treatment, because the side effects pose an unacceptable risk.

✔ Can take a wait-and-see approach. Some folks with less-advanced disease may want to wait a few years to see if better treatments come along. Your doctor will still check your liver enzyme/function tests regularly and may recommend a repeated biopsy (see Chapter 7 for more on these tests). The future of hep C medications is covered in the section "Researching Future Medical Treatments," later in this chapter.

The seriousness of the side effects causes some people to consider other options for therapy (see Chapter 10).

Testing for virus and liver disease

To start the evaluation process, your doctor will perform many of the virus and liver blood tests that I cover in Chapters 6 and 7. Here are some of the medical guidelines for determining who'd most benefit from peginterferon plus ribavirin treatment (assuming that you don't have any factors against treatment, as described in the section "Outlining factors that rule out treatment," later in this chapter).

Everyone who's treated must have hep C virus RNA in their blood. Treatment is usually recommended if you have chronic hepatitis C with clear evidence of liver disease — your liver biopsy shows some fibrosis. Treatment is recommended on a case-by-case basis if:

✔ You have absent to mild liver disease — liver biopsy showing no or mild fibrosis.

✔ You have acute hepatitis C (early infection).

✔ You're co-infected with HIV.

✔ You're under 18 years of age.

✔ You have decompensated cirrhosis. (End-stage liver disease must be treated at a liver transplant center.)

✔ You're a liver transplant recipient.

Your doctor will also look for certain factors that may lessen your success with interferon treatment, including high hep C viral load (see Chapter 6), high levels of iron (see Chapter 7), or fatty deposits in the liver (see Chapters 7 and 11).

You and your doctor must weigh the danger of your liver disease against the problems that might ensue with peginterferon plus ribavirin treatment, which may be greater for folks with HIV, end-stage liver disease, or a liver transplant.

Considering genotype

Your doctor will test your blood to see what type of genotype your virus is (see Chapter 6 for more on genotypes). The most common genotype in the United States and Canada is genotype 1. Genotypes 2 and 3 are the next most common. The genotype is a major factor in determining how well and how quickly peginterferon plus ribavirin therapy rids your body of hep C:

✔ **Genotype 1:** The success rate for genotype 1 is about 50 percent, and a 48-week treatment is required. Because the chances are about 50–50 that you might go through a rigorous treatment protocol and not eliminate the virus, your doctor will probably perform a biopsy and discuss with you the risks and benefits of treatment.

✔ **Genotype 2 or 3:** When patients are treated with peginterferon with ribavirin, the success rate is 70 to 80 percent. Some doctors, after finding out that you have genotype 2 or 3, will recommend treatment and may not even suggest you go through the risk of a liver biopsy. The treatment time for these genotypes is also shorter (24 weeks). The most-recent studies show (for reasons that aren't yet clear) that genotype 3 infection may cause more fatty change in the liver, which may also influence the response to treatment.

There haven't been as many clinical trials to see how people with other genotypes (4 through 6) respond to treatment, though it appears to be in the range between genotypes 1 and 2.

Reviewing your health

If you have one of these preexisting health conditions, your doctor will want to make sure that these illnesses are under control before starting treatment:

- ✔ Anemia
- ✔ Autoimmune disease
- ✔ Heart disease
- ✔ Depression
- ✔ Psychosis

Treatment might worsen these illnesses, so you and your doctor must decide whether treatment is worth the risk.

Outlining factors that rule out treatment

You won't be treated for hepatitis C if the following apply to you:

- ✔ You're allergic to one of the components.
- ✔ You or your partner is currently pregnant or plans to become pregnant within time of treatment and six months afterward. The treatment is likely to cause birth defects or death of an unborn child.

Most doctors also won't treat you if you're actively using intravenous drugs or you're a heavy alcohol user. Further, they expect you to be clean and/or sober for at least six months before starting treatment.

Doctors prefer not to treat patients with an active addiction for these reasons:

- ✔ You could reinfect yourself with hepatitis C through your drug use or cause serious liver disease through alcohol use.
- ✔ You're considered less likely to be able to deal with the rigors of treatment: taking your medication correctly and regularly, attending doctor's visits, and reporting any side effects. If you don't take your medication properly, the effectiveness is decreased (see the section "Assessing your commitment," later in the chapter).

Even if you give up your addiction, you still need strong support, because the side effects of peginterferon and ribavirin could cause a relapse of addiction. (See the section "Understanding the Side Effects," later in this chapter, to see what to expect.) If you're a heavy alcohol or intravenous drug user and want treatment, give up your addiction (for helpful resources, see Chapter 12), and make sure to have a support system in place to help you through the ups and downs of treatment.

Doctors differ in the way they treat former or present addicts and heavy alcohol users. See Chapter 5 for tips on finding a doctor you can work with.

Finding the right time

Timing is everything in hep C treatment. It's a consideration in terms of getting treated in time to stop your disease in its tracks and in selecting a time in your personal life that's conducive to treatment.

If your lifestyle is too hectic to handle the demands and complications of treatment, your doctor may suggest that you wait until things calm down to be treated. Family or work demands can make timing your treatment difficult. And don't forget other demands, such as school — if you're currently finishing your college degree, for example, your doctor may want to wait till you graduate. (Health insurance is also an issue, because most folks need to be working or in school to receive insurance to cover the medical bills. See Chapter 16 for tips on dealing with work and financial issues.)

During parts of your treatment, you may not be able to work or take care of yourself, let alone be the primary caretaker of your family. Your doctor will want to check that you have a support system to make sure you can deal with the side effects.

Assessing your commitment

In addition to testing to see whether you're a good medical candidate before starting you on hep C drug treatment, your doctor will make sure that you'll follow through on your commitment to the treatment (*patient compliance,* in med speak). You need to consider your answers to the following questions:

> ✔ Are you serious about starting and finishing the hepatitis C medication even if you have some side effects? If you become depressed or have any other serious side effects, will you discuss that with your doctor immediately?

✔ Are you willing to use two methods of birth control for the duration of the treatment, which could be almost a year? (See Chapter 18 for more on birth control and hep C.)

✔ Will you show up for the regular office or lab visits to have blood taken?

Speak to your family before starting treatment. You'll need their support to help you deal with side effects (see Chapter 14). Speak to your partner about the issues of birth control.

Understanding the Side Effects

Before you start drug treatment, you may not have any symptoms, and your chronic hepatitis C may be relatively silent. When you begin peginterferon plus ribavirin therapy, however, you're likely to have some side effects. You may need medical intervention to manage side effects, and you may even need to stop working for a while.

Many people feel that trying to eradicate their hep C infection is worth the risk of side effects and complications. This decision, like all medical decisions, is intensely personal. I suggest that you read about side effects here and check out the information about the specific medication your doctor recommends from the pharmaceutical companies (see Chapter 22 for contact information) before starting the treatment so that you're well aware of what to expect.

Each of you will respond differently to the treatment. Here's some general self-care advice that you'll probably hear from many sources (including your doctor) and elsewhere in this book that will help tame some side effects:

✔ Try to drink between 8 and 10 glasses of water or another clear liquid (like apple juice) every day. If you have diarrhea or vomiting, drink more liquid.

✔ Try light exercise and stress relievers (see Chapter 13), which can help with anxiety, fatigue, headaches, and so on.

✔ Follow the suggestions for good nutrition outlined in Chapter 11. Avoid alcohol, high levels of caffeine, and sugar.

✔ Try injecting before bedtime so that you avoid some side effects during the day.

Here are more common side effects from peginterferon plus ribavirin treatment and some self-help tips you can try:

- ✔ **Fatigue:** Try getting to sleep early each night, and take naps early in the day.

- ✔ **Flu-like symptoms:** These symptoms include headaches and muscle aches, fever, and chills. Speak to your doctor about taking acetaminophen for any pain or discomfort.

- ✔ **Gastrointestinal symptoms:** These symptoms include nausea, vomiting, lack of appetite, and weight loss. Avoid greasy, fried foods. Eat small healthy meals, even if you're not hungry (see Chapter 11 for nutrition advice).

- ✔ **Emotional/mental problems:** Symptoms include insomnia, anxiety or irritability, and depression. I provide some tips on getting to sleep at night in Chapter 21. You may need medication or benefit from talking to a mental health professional (see Chapter 14).

- ✔ **Hair loss (alopecia):** Avoid hair coloring, permanents, curling irons, and so on. Use a gentle shampoo.

- ✔ **Pain or redness at the site of infection:** Use a different injection site each time, and try ice before injecting.

- ✔ **Itchiness:** Avoid hot water in baths and showers, and use gentle soaps and moisturizers.

You may need to see other types of healthcare professionals and use other drugs to help you deal with side effects. Some folks practice complementary and alternative medicine to help them deal with side effects. See Chapter 10 for more information.

Some side effects of the antiviral treatment can be serious or even life threatening. Possible side effects can cause problems with every system of your body, including your brain, eyes, skin, heart, blood, kidneys, and immune system. Read more about potential side effects in the product literature supplied by the pharmaceutical manufacturers or on their Web sites. Though serious side effects may be less common or even rare, they do happen.

Your doctor will monitor your health regularly, but you need to report any unusual or serious symptoms. Keep the following information in mind:

- ✔ Side effects from interferon tend to occur in the beginning of treatment and will get better with time, but make sure to tell your doctor about any side effects.

✔ Don't stop taking the medication without speaking to your doctor. Taking the meditation consistently is crucial to its effectiveness.

✔ Your doctor can always decrease your dose or help manage your side effects with other medications.

✔ If the peginterferon plus ribavirin therapy is causing life-threatening complications, your doctor of course will stop treatment.

Tell your doctor immediately if you have any of the following:

✔ Problems with your thyroid disease or diabetes

✔ Shortness of breath

✔ Chest pain

Responding to Treatment

The purpose of the antiviral treatment is to eliminate the hepatitis C virus in your body. Your doctor will check your response to treatment by measuring your:

✔ **Virologic response:** A *virologic response* means your virus load is either undetectable or has dropped significantly. Before, during, and after treatment, your blood will be checked for virus RNA (quantitative or qualitative RNA assay, described in Chapter 7). The following are the different times your virologic response is measured:

- **Early virologic response (EVR):** Twelve weeks after the start of treatment.

- **End-of-treatment virologic response (ETR):** End of treatment.

- **Sustained virologic response (SVR):** Six months after treatment ends.

The goal of treatment is to have a sustained virologic response where hep C RNA becomes undetectable for years after treatment.

✔ **Liver enzyme levels:** Another measurement of the success of antiviral therapy is its ability to bring your ALT and other liver enzyme/function test levels to "normal" levels (see Chapter 7 for discussion of these tests).

Following up a sustained virologic response: Is it a cure?

If you've finished treatment, and your doctor congratulates you with the news that you have a sustained virologic response (shortened as SVR, or sustained response), you may wonder what comes next. At this point, moving forward, most folks remain free of detectable virus and have a much-decreased risk of developing serious liver disease. This is the point at which your doctor might say you are cured. You deserve a celebration after the challenges you've gone through with drug treatment for so many months. I bet you feel better, too, with many of the symptoms of interferon treatment and your hep C disease eliminated.

Speak with your doctor about your results and what they mean in terms of your long-term health. At this point, all medical evidence suggests that sustained responders eradicate their virus for years. You must continue your medical visits to check that your liver function doesn't worsen and that the hep C virus has not returned.

To keep yourself healthy, continue to practice good nutrition (see Chapter 11), and keep your body, mind, and spirit fine-tuned (see Chapter 13). You're not protected from future infection with hepatitis C virus, so make sure to avoid situations in which hep C can be transmitted (see Chapter 2).

Looking at options for nonresponders or relapsers

If you still have elevated ALT levels or hep C viral RNA after drug treatment, you're considered to be a *nonresponder*. If you've responded to drug treatment and then become a nonresponder when off the medication, you're considered to be a *relapser*. It can be very depressing to be in one of these categories after going through the rigors of interferon treatment.

One bright note is that you're not alone, and medical researchers are actively looking for ways to help you.

Your liver doctor will know of current options that are suitable for you. She might suggest consensus interferon (Infergen; see the "Defining interferon" section, earlier in the chapter). You could consider joining a clinical trial of a new medication (see the sidebar "Participating in clinical trials" in this chapter).

Hepatitis C doctors are conscientious and creative about finding ways to help their patients, and you may come across other forms of interferon that are infrequently used to treat people who don't respond to the interferons listed in Table 8-1.

Another option is to consider visiting an alternative practitioner, such as an acupuncturist or herbalist, to see whether any of those treatments can help you. Alternative and complementary medical approaches are discussed in Chapter 10.

Researching Future Medical Treatments

Expect to see new developments in the next years and decades as bench work in the laboratory turns into clinical trials, which turn into new treatment protocols. Here are some things to watch for:

- ✓ **Variations on interferon and ribavirin treatment:** Down the road, this therapy may offer the following:
  - Different dosing regimes
  - Different ways to take the drugs
  - Modifications beyond pegylation for interferon and modifications of ribavirin that increase their effectiveness and reduce side effects
  - Use of additional agents to decrease side effects
- ✓ **New protocols or drugs for special populations:** Studies are underway in children, African Americans, Latinos, women, and people who don't respond to or can't take peginterferon plus ribavirin.
- ✓ **New drugs:** Medicines of the future may be able to:
  - Target specific areas of hep C virus replication
  - Help the immune system fight the hep C virus

See Chapter 3 to read about hep C virus replication and the immune response to hep C (especially inflammation). Future treatments will probably consist of a "cocktail" of drugs that fight hep C infection in different ways.

Participating in clinical trials

Before a new drug becomes available, it first goes through testing in clinical trials. Trials also look at different aspects of hepatitis C disease and treatment in different types of people. You might consider participating in a trial if:

✔ Conventional treatment with pegylated interferon and ribavirin hasn't worked for you.

✔ You have late-stage cirrhosis or liver cancer.

Or you just might be interested in contributing to scientific research. To find out about clinical trials, speak to your doctor, local hospital, and support groups for hep C. They can give you information on the trials so that you're well informed before you give your consent to the trial. Make sure to consider the risks and benefits of the treatment.

You can find out the basics about clinical trials and find a list of hepatitis C clinical trials by checking out www.clinicaltrials.gov, which is produced by the U.S. National Institutes of Health. Many of the resources in Chapter 22 also have information on hepatitis C clinical trials.

Treating Hepatitis C Symptoms

Perhaps you haven't tried treatment, and you're looking for other ways to deal with your hepatitis C symptoms. Or maybe you've tried treatment, and it hasn't worked for you (see the "Looking at options for nonresponders or relapsers" section, earlier in the chapter). Even if you try self-help techniques, such as modifying your diet and stress relief, to help relieve symptoms, you may still have problems and need medication. Some folks also find relief with complementary and alternative medicine treatments.

Your doctor can prescribe medication to help you with side effects and symptoms (see Chapter 4 for a list of symptoms).

In this section, I briefly list some medications, home remedies, and other treatments your doctor may suggest for problems associated with different types of hepatitis C disease.

Don't take any medication or herbal remedy (whether it's prescribed or over the counter) without first checking with your doctor. Make sure that your liver doctor is aware of all medications you're taking. I discuss the possible toxicity of medications in Chapter 12.

Each time you get a refill or new prescription, double-check the medication. Although unlikely, mistakes do happen:

- ✔ Make sure the drug name and dosage on the label match what you're expecting, based on what the doctor told you or what you're used to getting.

- ✔ If you switch brands or switch to a generic, double-check with the pharmacist if the pills look different to you.

- ✔ Add the name and dosage of this drug and the drug information leaflet that comes with your prescription to your hep C notebook (see Chapter 5 for more info on this notebook).

Chronic hepatitis

If you have chronic hepatitis, you may suffer none or many symptoms of the disease (which I discuss in Chapter 4). I don't have enough space in this book to list all the treatments for all these symptoms, but here are the most common problems:

- ✔ **Pain, muscle aches, and headaches:** Each type of painkiller for these symptoms has a list of side effects that may affect your hepatitis C, so please consult your doctor before taking any over-the-counter pain medication. Acetaminophen (Tylenol) in low doses is commonly prescribed for headaches and muscle aches.

- ✔ **Depression:** The cause of depression may be the hepatitis C or your drug treatment. Your doctor may prescribe an anti-depressant or refer you to a mental health professional (see Chapter 14), especially if you have a history of depression and are taking peginterferon plus ribavirin medication, which can increase or cause depression.

- ✔ **Itchiness:** This condition, also called pruritis, may occur if you have jaundice or as a side effect of medication. Your doctor probably will suggest not using water that is too hot in your bath or shower, trying oatmeal baths, and using moisturizers.

  Scratching may not relieve your itch, and you may scratch so much that you develop a bacterial infection of the skin.

  If you are still itchy, see your doctor to discuss medications for relief. Your doctor may prescribe a drug called cholestyramine, which blocks bile acids and can relieve itching. Other drugs used are antihistamines, antibiotics, or even sedatives.

- ✔ **Insomnia and other sleep problems:** Lack of sleep can contribute to fatigue and other symptoms of hepatitis C (see the tips for good sleep in Chapter 21). If you need help from your doctor, she may be able to prescribe a medication to help that doesn't hurt your liver. Don't be tempted to use alcohol or other drugs, which could hurt your liver (see Chapter 12).

✔ **Nausea and stomach disorders:** Your doctor may suggest changes in your diet or eating habits to help your digestion, but if those changes don't work, medications are also available to help with specific problems.

Complications of cirrhosis

Cirrhosis occurs with extensive scarring (fibrosis) of the liver. As your liver may not be able to function adequately, symptoms can be severe or life threatening. *Compensated cirrhosis* means that your liver can still function even with scarring. *Decompensated cirrhosis* is another name for end-stage liver disease, which results in liver failure unless you can get a liver transplant. See Chapter 4 for a discussion of progression of hep C disease and Chapter 9 for information about liver transplants.

Here is an overview of medical treatment for common complications of cirrhosis:

✔ **Ascites:** Treatment for ascites (fluid accumulation in the abdomen) may be a combination of bed rest, a salt-restricted diet (see Chapter 11), diuretics to eliminate fluids, and antibiotics to treat infections. Your doctor may also remove the fluid for examination and relief of discomfort.

✔ **Encephalopathy:** Cirrhosis can cause brain problems such as confusion, personality changes, or even a coma. See your doctor at any signs of confusion to avoid developing the more dangerous stage of coma. Treatment involves reducing your levels of protein; switching to vegetable sources of protein (see Chapter 11 for tips); and using the drug called lactulose, which is a sugary syrup that works well for many people. You also may need an antibiotic treatment.

✔ **Variceal bleeding:** To reduce portal hypertension and decrease the chance of bleeding as a result of cirrhosis, your doctor may prescribe beta-blocker drugs. Some surgical techniques may also be used if you develop this serious complication.

✔ **Tendency to bleed:** If your liver is no longer clotting properly, don't participate in contact sports or other activities with a high risk of bleeding. Don't take drugs with blood-thinning activity (such as aspirin and ibuprofen).

Although these symptoms can be managed by your doctor, liver transplantation is the medical "cure" for cirrhosis that has become decompensated, a condition that is also called end-stage liver disease (see Chapter 4).

Liver cancer

For people with primary liver cancer (hepatocellular carcinoma), treatments are surgery to remove the liver tumor (resection) or to remove the entire liver (liver transplant). Traditional chemotherapy and radiation generally aren't used for treatment. Pain relievers and other drugs are used to relieve any symptoms of the cancer.

Chapter 9

Getting a New Liver

● ●

In This Chapter

▶ Deciding whether you qualify for a transplant

▶ Going to a transplant center for evaluation

▶ Getting onto a waiting list

▶ Having transplant surgery

▶ Caring for yourself and your new liver

● ●

*H*ere's the good news: Most people with hep C don't need a liver transplant. Here's some more good news: If you have end-stage liver disease or liver cancer, a transplant can provide a new lease on life. The not-so-good news is that there aren't enough donor livers for everyone who needs one. Folks with liver disease and their family and friends frequently become advocates for organ donation.

When your doctor determines that you may need a new liver, you go onto a waiting list. Getting placed on this list requires evaluation by a transplant team. At that point, you're entered into the organ donation system, which directs donor livers to the most needy transplant candidates. Lifelong aftercare and medication are necessary to keep your new liver in tiptop shape.

Liver transplantation is nothing short of a miracle provided by the donor with the aid of the transplant team. Success stories are common, but if a transplant isn't on your horizon, feel free to skip over this chapter, with the knowledge that you can always check it out later. But should you or a loved one face the prospects of a liver transplant, this chapter provides an introduction to the process and helps you find even more information.

Meeting the Folks Who Need a New Liver

Although most people with hepatitis C don't need a liver transplant, hep C accounts for 40 percent of all liver transplants in the United States today. (Other causes or types of liver disease and sudden liver failure account for the remaining liver transplants.)

Most of the hep C folks who need a liver transplant have struggled with chronic hepatitis C disease for years. Their disease has progressed into one of these irreversible life-threatening conditions:

- **End-stage liver disease:** This condition is also called decompensated cirrhosis.

- **Primary liver cancer:** Also referred to as hepatocellular carcinoma, this is cancer that starts in the liver and is *not* from cancer that originates elsewhere in the body.

In Chapter 4, I describe the different symptoms and diseases that can come with the hepatitis C virus, including the illnesses in the preceding list.

Preventing death due to imminent liver failure or liver cancer is the reason to transplant a liver. Without a liver transplant, end-stage liver disease will result in liver failure and death. Liver cancer that isn't removed by transplantation or by another surgical technique, called *resection,* will also result in eventual death as the cancer spreads to other parts of the body.

Traveling the Trail to a Transplant

Your primary care or specialist physician takes the first step toward a transplant for you by referring you to a transplant center after determining that you need a new liver. You may have been under a specialist's care for years and only recently developed more serious symptoms or liver cancer.

In the United States, the United Network for Organ Sharing (UNOS) coordinates the procurement, matching, and placement of all donated organs by managing the Organ Procurement and Transplantation Network (OPTN). (For more information on all aspects of organ transplant, see the UNOS Web site at www. unos.org.)

The United States is divided into 11 geographic regions (each with multiple states) that contain 59 local *organ procurement organizations* (OPOs), which manage the physical acquisition and delivery of the organs. Each local OPO has individual transplant centers, which are housed at individual hospitals.

If your transplant center qualifies you as a potential liver recipient, your name is submitted to UNOS, which adds your name to the national pool — or list — of folks waiting for livers.

Choosing a transplant center

More than 200 hospitals perform liver transplants in the United States. In Canada, approximately 28 hospitals perform transplants. Depending on where you live, you may have a choice of centers. If so, consider the following factors:

- ✔ **Experience of the liver transplant team:** How many operations does it perform yearly? How long has the team been doing liver transplants?

- ✔ **Waiting list:** What's the average wait for a liver at this center? Each region and each transplant center has different average wait times because of differences in the number of donors or number of people on the waiting list.

- ✔ **Geographic proximity:** You and your personal support team must be close to the hospital to get to surgery quickly and be able to attend aftercare.

- ✔ **Cost of surgery and recovery:** This amount varies by location and individual hospital. Your health insurance may be affiliated with or work better at certain hospitals. Ask your health plan administrator or the financial administrator of the transplant center for specifics regarding your insurance coverage.

If you or someone you care about needs a transplant, you can start to fill in the blanks by speaking to your liver specialist and the transplant coordinator at individual centers. General information is available on the Web, and you can search for information on the different transplant centers. Also check out these sources:

- ✔ **In the United States:** Check out the Transplant Living Web site (www.transplantliving.org), a comprehensive and informative site from UNOS (www.unos.org), the organization that administers the organ transplant network in the United States. Also take a look at www.ustranplant.org.

✔ **In Canada:** Visit the Organ and Tissue Information Site from
Health Canada (www.hc-sc.gc.ca/english/organand
tissue). Each province has separate policies for liver transplantation, so you must check with your local health authority
for information.

Enrolling at the center

At the transplant center, you'll be evaluated by the transplant
team, which is made up of experts in hepatology, surgery, psychia-
try, social services, nutrition, cardiology, and finances. The goal is
to identify people who most desperately need a new liver.

A nurse is assigned as your transplant team coordinator and serves
as your primary point of contact during the preliminary evaluation
(and throughout the transplant process). Doctors examine the cause
of your liver failure and your health in general. You also see a psychiatrist and social worker to develop the support needed before
and after surgery. Because of the high cost of transplant surgery and
necessary lifelong medication, a financial officer helps you organize
your benefits. And a nutritionist helps make sure that your diet
provides you the nourishment you need before and after transplant.

Enrolling at a transplant center doesn't mean that you're on the official waiting list for a liver. Your transplant center will first perform
certain tests to determine your eligibility. Then your transplant
coordinator will tell you whether you're on the list.

MELDing scores

Your transplant center will perform certain tests to determine your
eligibility and placement on the national waiting list managed by
UNOS. A standardized score called *MELD* (model for end-stage liver
disease) is calculated for adults, and a score called *PELD* (pediatric
end-stage liver disease) is figured for those under 18. These scores
aim to measure how likely a potential recipient is to die while waiting for a transplant.

The MELD scores are based on results from these laboratory tests
(which you can read more about in Chapter 7):

✔ **Bilirubin levels in the blood:** A measure of bilirubin levels
indicates whether the liver is clearing this toxin (which causes
jaundice) and making bile.

✔ **INR/PT (international normalized ratio/prothrombin time):**
This test measures the liver's production of blood-clotting
factors.

✔ **Creatinine levels:** This test is used as a measure of kidney function, which deteriorates as a result of liver failure.

The PELD score is determined by using the three MELD factors (bilirubin, INR/PR, and creatinine) and also albumin levels, failure to grow (measured by gender, height, and weight), and age at time of listing.

The data are entered into a computer, and a mathematical formula produces the MELD/PELD score, which can range from 6 to 40. Anything over 40 is called 40, because this is the highest category. The higher MELD/PELD scores represent more serious illness.

Scientists and medical doctors developed the MELD/PELD scores as the most accurate way to access need for a liver transplant. Like all rules, there are exceptions, and your transplant center can apply for more points in certain severe medical situations — or even for a more crucial category called Liver Status 1. Because the need for liver transplants is so urgent, rules are constantly being reevaluated to provide the fairest method of organ allocation possible.

While you're on the waiting list, regular retesting is a must to keep your certified place on the list — or to put you at a higher place due to worsening condition (see Table 9-1). Your doctor and transplant center will advise you on how often you need to get retested. Keep up with your testing, or you may lose your chance for a transplant.

Table 9-1	Waiting List Recertification Times
Classification	*Time Frame for Recertification*
Liver Status 1	Every 7 days
MELD/PELD 25+	Every 7 days
MELD/PELD 19–24	Every 30 days
MELD/PELD 11–18	Every 90 days
MELD/PELD 10 or less	Every year

Facing disqualification — and taking action

Unfortunately, getting a new liver isn't an option for everyone who needs one. Even if you have a failing liver or liver cancer, some situations may disqualify you for a transplant.

If you fall into one of the following categories, discuss your options with your doctor. She might prescribe medications to help ease any pain or slow your cancer.

✔ Existing heart, lung, or kidney disease that would complicate your ability to survive the surgery and/or post-transplant

✔ Liver cancer that is too big (one tumor over 5 centimeters or multiple tumors that are over 3 centimeters) or has spread to other organs

Evidence of *current* alcohol or intravenous drug use may disqualify you from consideration. Use of some drugs that were formerly disapproved of (methadone and marijuana) may now be accepted in some clinics. See Chapter 12 for information on alcohol or drug addiction and a list of resources for overcoming addiction.

Inability to pay for either the surgery or the lifelong medication needed to keep the transplant healthy afterward can also disqualify you for a transplant. But help is available.

You may need help paying for a transplant and the associated lifelong medication. The financial administrator and social worker at the transplant center may help you find ways to finance the transplant and aftercare.

Transplant Living has an excellent list of U.S. resources to contact that include charitable organizations, Medicare, and prescription drug assistance plans. Use these general ideas to obtain necessary funding in other countries. Go to www.transplantliving.org/ beforethetransplant. Within the "Financing a Transplant Section," you'll find "Financial Resources Directory." Family and friends can help by contacting these agencies on your behalf and perhaps even organizing a fund-raising event.

Allocating organs

Unless you use a living donor, you probably face a wait, along with people all over the country, between the time of listing and receipt of a transplant.

When a liver becomes available through a sudden brain death, the local OPO is in charge of safely obtaining the organ (procurement) and informing UNOS of the available liver (see descriptions of these organizations in the "Traveling the Trail to a Transplant" section, earlier in the chapter). UNOS uses a computer analysis of people who are waiting for a transplant to decide where the liver should go. UNOS has a 17-page document with rules for allocation of livers. I've generalized the rules here:

- ✔ **MELD score (or Liver Status 1):** Liver Status 1 gets priority over the MELD score. The higher your MELD score, the higher on the list you are.

- ✔ **Age:** All things being equal in scores, pediatric cases precede adults.

- ✔ **Geographic proximity:** Time is of the essence when getting an organ to a potential recipient, so the transplant centers closest in location to the donor organ are given preference. Local centers have priority, followed by regional and then national.

- ✔ **Matching of donor and recipient:** It's best when donor and recipient have compatible blood types (though not necessary in some emergency Liver Status 1 cases). Also, size may be a factor, because a large liver can be too big for a small person (but a smaller liver can grow inside a larger person).

In cases in which all other factors match, time on the waiting list may be factored in. Otherwise, disease severity takes priority over time waiting on the list. When a center is offered an organ, it has an hour or less to notify the UNOS center that it'll use the organ. For that reason, the transplant center must be able to reach you at all times. Your center may require you to have a cell phone or beeper or to stay within a certain geographic area while waiting. The closer you live to the center, the better the chances that the organ will be in excellent condition when it is put into your body.

Contrary to the urban myth that states that fame and fortune will move you higher up the list, UNOS states, "Race, gender, religion, socio-economic status, or personal/behavioral history are not taken into account in organ allocation policy."

Waiting, waiting, waiting

The shortage of donor organs creates an urgent problem for which the waiting list is the present solution. Waiting for a transplant can be stressful for you and your family. You're facing a life-threatening illness and the uncertainty about if and when you'll receive a transplant.

Reaching out for support, practicing stress management, and aiming for a positive outlook will help you and your family. Here are some additional tips to consider:

✔ Look for a support group at your transplant center — remember that others are also on the waiting list.

✔ Though it's easier said than done, try to reduce other sources of stress in your life, and develop positive and effective ways of dealing with stress. (I include lots of ideas for stress reduction in Chapter 13 and tips for dealing with emotions in Chapter 14.)

✔ You may need to watch your salt, iron, and protein intake. Follow the suggestions of your doctors and nutritionists, and improve your diet and nutrition (see Chapter 11).

✔ Have your bags packed and ready to go! Be ready to go to the hospital when that call arrives.

You can try to find another center within your region or in a different region that may have shorter waiting times. Registering at more than one center is acceptable at most centers, as long as you notify all parties. Make sure to check for coverage of the different centers with your insurance company.

Discuss the logistics of a transplant with your family and extended support group. You will need them when the call for a liver comes.

Transplanting the Liver

Liver transplantation has a high success rate. The national one-year survival rates are 85 to 86 percent, and five-year survival rates are more than 70 percent for end-stage liver disease and 50 percent for liver cancer.

During the operation, you may need a blood transfusion. Speak to your doctor if you want to donate your own blood ahead of time.

You may receive two types of transplant:

✔ **Whole organ donation:** This liver comes from a patient who is declared brain-dead (see the sidebar "Conquering myths about the gift of life," later in this chapter). The liver is extracted, preserved on ice, transported to the hospital, and transplanted within 12 to 18 hours.

✔ **Partial liver transplant:** This liver can come from a live or a brain-dead donor. Either a piece of liver from a healthy person or part of a liver from a deceased person is transplanted. Segments of the liver will regenerate into a fully functioning liver. Living donors may be relatives or unrelated as long as the blood type matches.

Conquering myths about the gift of life

More than 85,000 people are waiting for donation of organs. Sadly, some die before they receive an organ. Here are some of the common misconceptions that keep people from donating.

Myth: Brain death is not really death.

Fact: Death of the body occurs when either the heart or the brain stops working. Most familiar is heart death: when the heart stops beating. Brain death means the brain has stopped functioning and never will function again. This is different from a brain coma or vegetative state.

At brain death, a short window of time exists in which death is certain, but the other organs are functional while the body is on support systems.

Myth: If you're listed as an organ donor, emergency care workers will not try to save your life.

Fact: This common fear is untrue. Healthcare workers don't stop trying to save your life until you are dead. If you're declared brain-dead, your family will be contacted about organ donation.

Myth: If my driver's license says that I am an organ donor, or I have an organ donor card, that is enough.

Fact: Tell your family your wishes, in addition to having documentation about dona-tion. Medical staffs always discuss donation with your family.

In a donation from a living person, the donor faces her own risk from the major surgery to remove part of her liver.

Transplant surgery is complex. Your diseased liver must be care-fully removed, with connections to vessels and ducts carefully severed. The new organ is then reattached to the vessels and ducts. You'll spend some time in the intensive care unit after surgery and days to weeks in the hospital.

Your transplant center will let you know if they perform alternative types of transplants to enable them to decrease your waiting time. Because of the shortage of donor livers, some centers perform these types of transplants:

- ✔ Two partial-liver donations from one organ
- ✔ Transplants with older or hepatitis C–infected donor livers
- ✔ Live liver donations

Although these procedures might not be commonly performed right now, further studies and improvements by transplant surgeons will allow such techniques to be used to maximize the number of people who can be helped with the limited supply of donor livers.

Living with a New Liver

Maintaining a foreign organ in your body requires good healthcare. Your body will see the new liver as "foreign" (read about this aspect of the immune system in Chapter 3). To maintain your liver, you need to:

✔ Take medication for the rest of your life to avoid rejection of your new organ. Talk to your doctor about how to manage the side effects of these essential drugs:

- Cortisone-like drugs may cause fluid retention and puffiness, and may trigger diabetes and osteoporosis.

- Cyclosporine, an immunosuppressive drug, can lead to high blood pressure, unwanted body hair, or kidney damage.

- FK-506, another immunosuppressant, can cause headaches, tremors, diarrhea, and kidney problems.

✔ Avoid exposure to infections because your immune system is weakened by your immunosuppressive medication. Some steps to take in this regard include avoiding sick people and large crowds and practicing safer sex, especially with new partners.

✔ See your doctor regularly for tests to make sure you're not rejecting your new liver.

✔ Eat a balanced diet, and reduce your salt intake to avoid water retention (see Chapter 11 for more on nutrition).

✔ The hep C virus will probably return to your liver, so follow the suggestions for good health outlined in Part III. The exact location of hidden hepatitis virus isn't known, but studies have found that transplanted livers do become infected. Other studies are looking at the feasibility of antiviral treatment for transplant recipients. This therapy is tricky, however, because interferon, for example, increases the immune response, and cyclosporine decreases the immune response.

After a transplant, life will return to something near normal for you. Within 6 to 12 months after surgery, you may resume physical and sexual activities, as desired. Continue to get support from your doctors, transplant team, and support groups for any anxieties that accompany these major life changes. Check out www.transweb.org for info on living with a transplant from the patient's perspective.

Chapter 10

Looking at Types of Treatment: Western, Complementary, and Alternative Medicine

*Y*ou may become confused when you first investigate treatment options for hepatitis C. Your doctor recommends one thing, your sister suggests another, and you may find something else on the Web. How do you decide what to do? People may recommend one thing over another, but what is the evidence?

Before deciding on treatment, make sure to have results from virus and liver testing (see Chapters 6 and 7) and a doctor who understands hepatitis C and liver disease (see Chapter 5). You also need to know what stage of the disease you have. If your biopsy shows no fibrosis, and your ALT levels (which I explain in Chapter 7) are normal, you'll make different decisions than if you have advanced fibrosis and the early stages of cirrhosis (see Chapter 4).

You also need to assess your financial situation in terms of your health plan coverage and what personal funds you have, if any, to pursue treatment not covered by your health plan.

In this chapter, I describe the conventional, complementary, and alternative treatments for hep C and give you ways to do further research. You can find detailed information on the current best conventional medical treatment in Chapter 8. Chapters 11, 12, and 13 give information on lifestyle changes that will also help you heal from hep C.

You're the one choosing which treatments to pursue. I recommend that you read each of the sections on treatment, consult your doctor, and talk with your support network before making a decision.

Considering the Evidence

This section is for folks with inquisitive minds — those who want to know the different options available. I tell you how to find information on hep C treatments and what to look for.

Gathering information

When comparing different hepatitis C treatments, you'll have to evaluate the information you get. The first question to ask yourself is, who's providing this information? You also need to ask yourself what the motivation is in promoting treatments for hepatitis C. Here are common sources of information that you may encounter:

- **Your healthcare practitioner:** Speak to your doctor, who'll advise you based on his knowledge and experience with hepatitis C treatment, including what he has learned from his education and in the process of treating the people with hep C. I include a list of questions to ask your practitioner in Chapter 5. You may want to speak to more than one doctor.

- **The Internet:** The Web is filled with information that varies from incredibly useful to downright dangerous. You can find information on hep C treatment by checking out the links I give throughout this chapter, the rest of the book, and Chapter 22.

  When evaluating the evidence on a Web site, try to find out who's in charge of the site. One way to get this info is to go the home page or About Us page and see who produces the material and what bias the people or groups running the site may have. Government agencies, doctors and medical organizations, liver foundations or other hepatitis not-for-profit organizations, and even individuals with hepatitis C all run hep C sites.

  Remember that *anyone* can post information on the Internet, and designing a Web site to advertise products that claim to "cure" hepatitis C is relatively simple. Read information much more carefully when a site sells products. Find a reputable practitioner to advise you, and run the other way if you see words like *miraculous cure* and *amazing*.

✔ **Friends, family, and other people with hep C:** You may find people giving you their two cents' worth about treatment. People have opinions based on their personal experience or what they've heard from others. For example, if someone has a good result with acupuncture, she'll recommend it. If another person had her virus cleared with interferon treatment, she'll suggest you begin drug therapy. Just remember that this is *anecdotal* evidence, which means it works in that particular situation. Just because a treatment works for one person doesn't mean it'll work on you, although it may, so investigate further.

 If you're inclined to do your own research about all things medical, consider these resources for hep C medical info (in addition to the resources I include in Chapter 22, many of which have loads of information on clinical trials or medical studies):

✔ **Entrez PubMed:** You can search for medical abstracts on this Web page, part of the National Library of Medicine. Go to www.ncbi.nlm.nih.gov/entrez.

✔ **The Clinical Care Options for Hepatitis Web page:** Go to www.clinicaloptions.com/hep. You must register (for free) to access this up-to-date information, which is written for doctors but available to everyone.

✔ **The HIV and hepatitis Web site:** Go to www.hivandhepatitis.com for excellent and updated information on hepatitis C. You can also ask questions about treatment: Just click on the "The Doctor Is In" link.

You may find yourself with gobs of information from medical studies or trials and wondering how you'll deal with this information. I suggest that you ask these questions about each study:

✔ **What's the date of the study?** In most cases, the more recent work is the most relevant.

✔ **How many people were treated?** The larger the study, the more applicable it is to lots of other people.

✔ **Did the study include people like you?** In other words, were they your gender, race, hep C virus status (high or low amounts of virus), and genotype?

✔ **Did the study use controls?** Studies that use controls (people who don't get the drug being tested) are more likely to get results that can be repeated.

Also, check out any information on how many people dropped out of the study because of side effects.

Don't forget to consult your hepatitis C doctor, who has had years of specialized training that helps put research into perspective.

Comparing different treatments

So much information is out there that people can be easily swayed by arguments about different types of evidence. When collecting evidence, write down the pros and cons of each treatment. Use the following list to start to gather information about any treatments you're considering. You can also use it to compare the relative merits of different treatments:

- ✔ Name of treatment
- ✔ Purpose of treatment
- ✔ Effectiveness of treatment
- ✔ Side effects
- ✔ Length of treatment time
- ✔ Cost of treatment
- ✔ Results of stopping treatment
- ✔ Related insurance coverage
- ✔ Other info I need to know

Many factors go into making decisions about which treatments are right for you. The rest of this chapter describes different types of conventional, alternative, and complementary treatments.

Describing Different Treatments for Hep C

Hepatitis C treatments aren't "one size fits all." Healing modes vary from pharmaceutical medications to acupuncture to herbal remedies. Staying open-minded about different choices will give you the best chance of finding the right treatment. The two general categories of treatments for hepatitis C are:

- ✔ **Conventional Western medicine:** Medicine taught in mainstream medical schools
- ✔ **Complementary and alternative medicine:** Medical practices from other cultures or belief systems

More people are now integrating their healthcare, using the best of Western medicine with the best of alternative practices. The formerly distinct line between conventional Western medicine and alternative medicines is becoming blurred because of these reasons:

- ✔ People with hepatitis C are using both types of treatments.

- ✔ Alternative treatments are undergoing rigorous tests for effectiveness and safety.

- ✔ Conventional healthcare workers are learning about and incorporating some aspects of alternative medicine.

- ✔ Alternative practitioners work cooperatively with conventional treatment and use the results of diagnostic tests (such as liver enzyme tests or liver biopsies) to confirm their own work.

Conventional Western medicine

The major type of medicine approved by health plans, hospitals, and doctors in the United States today is called conventional, or Western, medicine.

 Medical science aims to understand the cause of disease at a detailed level. Diseases are caused by individual genes or mutations within the gene; chemicals; or infectious agents, like the hepatitis C virus in combination with cofactors. Drugs are designed to stop the chain of events that lead to illness.

As I cover in Chapters 8 and 9, Western medicine uses a two-pronged approach to treat hepatitis C.

Drugs to treat hepatitis C and symptoms

The following are the types of drugs you'd use for hepatitis C:

- ✔ **Antiviral medicines:** These drugs seek to eliminate the hep C virus. The current best treatment is a combination of pegylated interferon and ribavirin, which I discuss in Chapter 8.

- ✔ **Medications to treat symptoms:** These drugs treat symptoms but don't eliminate the virus. For example, the drug lactulose is used to treat encephalopathy arising from cirrhosis (see Chapter 8).

- ✔ **Anticancer medications:** Chemotherapeutic agents haven't been very successful at helping people with liver cancer. But we can all hope that the future brings more effective and safe drugs for this type of cancer.

✔ **Antirejection medications:** These drugs, also known as immunosuppressive medications, allow a transplanted liver to thrive in your body (see Chapter 9 for more on transplants).

Surgery to treat liver disease

Here are the two ways that a skilled surgeon can treat liver cancer or end-stage liver disease with surgery:

✔ **Resection:** This term refers to the cutting away of liver tumors if you have liver cancer. Transplant surgery has a better longer-term success rate, but donor livers are in short supply.

✔ **Liver transplant:** Surgeons can transplant a whole liver or part of a donated liver in a person with liver failure (end-stage liver disease) or a person who's in certain stages of liver cancer.

Complementary and alternative medicine (CAM)

The term complementary and alternative medicine (CAM) is used to describe medical treatment that hasn't been part of conventional medical practice. The distinction between CAM and Western medicine is fading as more people choose to use both systems. The interest in CAM among many folks is a reflection of some dissatisfaction with conventional medical practice and/or the desire to try a different approach to their healthcare. The current trend is toward an integrated approach to healthcare, which encourages you to use the best of any treatment to get well.

Describing the components of CAM

More than 100 healing philosophies, approaches, and treatments are included in the term CAM. Here are some treatments that may be used as part of hepatitis C treatment:

✔ **Alternative medical systems:** These systems include traditional Chinese medicine (including acupuncture), ayurveda, homeopathy, and naturopathy, which I cover in the aptly named "Alternative Medical Systems" section, later in the chapter.

✔ **Biologically-based therapies:** Herbal medicine (see the "Herbal medicine" section, later in this chapter) and food and vitamin therapy are included in this category.

✔ **Mind-body techniques:** This category includes meditation, breathing, relaxation, and guided imagery, which I cover in Chapter 13.

✔ **Body-based therapies:** These treatments include the many types of massage, which is covered in Chapter 13.

✔ **Energy therapies:** Reiki and therapeutic touch are two types of treatments in this category, which I also cover in Chapter 13.

Differing ways of approaching health and medicine

Alternative medicine often views illness in a different way than conventional medicine does. Here are some general characteristics of alternative treatments and ways in which they may differ from Western medicine:

✔ **Your body, mind, and spirit are interconnected.** Increasingly, Western doctors realize the importance of stress and mood on illness, but spiritual matters are rarely discussed. CAM treatment is more likely to consider all parts of your being, including your mind and your spirit. The mind and body aren't seen as being separate entities but as intimately related.

✔ **All of your symptoms are considered at once.** A CAM practitioner looks at you as a whole. Western medicine frequently tells you that symptoms in different parts of the body aren't related, and you may be sent to visit different doctors to discuss different symptoms. A CAM practitioner is looking for a larger overriding theme (such as energy imbalance) to your illness that could explain lots of different symptoms.

With hepatitis C, your Western doctor will be interested in all your symptoms because they could be related to liver disease.

✔ **CAM treats your energy system.** Many CAM treatments believe that symptoms and disease are a byproduct of an energy disorder. By balancing or harmonizing your energy, the symptoms will disappear. CAM treatments differ in what they call the energy they work with. Chinese medicine calls it *qi* (chi). Other healing systems call it *vital energy* or *animating force.* Reiki brings in *universal energy* to heal you, and ayurvedic medicine calls it *prana.*

✔ **Natural products are used.** CAM treatments are based on the healing power of nature. Many Western treatments are derived from natural sources, though they're then synthetically produced. Interferon, for example, is a natural product of the body's immune system that is synthesized for use in hepatitis C treatment (see Chapter 8). CAM uses whole herbs or products from the herb itself.

✔ **Most treatments are unique for each person.** CAM treatments are more likely to be individually tailored for you. In general, Western medicine uses one major treatment for everyone with hepatitis C (peginterferon plus ribavirin), although scientists are looking for new treatments that will work for more people.

Considering the evidence

Although things are slowly changing, conventional medicine still hasn't widely embraced CAM treatments. The primary reason is the lack of scientific evidence for CAM's effectiveness and safety in treating disease. Here's a description of the evidence for the two types of treatment systems.

Conventional medicine for hep C

Many clinical trials have tested different types of interferon with and without ribavirin. These trials have led to a medical consensus on the current best treatment: the combination of pegylated interferon with ribavirin. Depending on your genotype, the treatment eliminates hep C virus in 50 to 80 percent of people treated. The U.S. Food and Drug Administration (FDA) has approved this and similar treatments for hep C.

More studies of different variations of treatments for hep C are ongoing. Newer, more effective, and ideally safer drug therapy will be available in the years to come. See Chapter 8 for more info on the conventional treatment of hep C.

CAM treatment for Hep C

Many CAM treatments were developed hundreds or thousands of years ago, before the use of statistics and clinical trials. Performing clinical trials with CAM treatments is more difficult, because clinical trials are expensive and CAM treatments are individually tailored, so finding a useful control group is difficult.

In response to the public interest on CAM, the U.S. National Institutes of Health (NIH) added a new center in 1998: the National Center for Complementary and Alternative Medicine (NCCAM), which you can read more about at www.nccam.nih.gov. The purpose of NCCAM and similar initiatives around the world is to increase the number of well-designed scientific studies on CAM treatments. As evidence builds for the safety and usefulness of any particular CAM, it becomes incorporated into conventional medicine.

Putting it all together

If you want firm FDA-approved treatments, go with conventional medicine. If you like the idea of alternative treatments and are willing to accept the lack of firm scientific evidence, go with CAM treatments. My advice is to take the best of both worlds instead of sticking with just one system of treatment. Many people take this approach to medicine, which has a new name: *integrated medicine.*

Having an optimistic placebo effect

When you really believe in your treatment, the chances of healing with that treatment are greater. Positive thinking is a powerful healer. Some critics of CAM say that its results are from the placebo effect, meaning that a certain percentage of people will get well from a treatment just because they believe the treatment will work. Wow, that's a confirmation of the power of the mind–body connection. Whatever treatment you use, make sure to believe in it, because whether it works on its own or whether it is the placebo effect doesn't really matter.

Here are two ways that you can integrate the different systems of health treatment:

✔ Use CAM treatments to help you deal with the side effects of Western peginterferon plus ribavirin treatment, but be sure to tell your Western medicine doctor.

✔ Use CAM treatments while you're waiting for new Western treatments to become available (all the while hoping that the CAM might be effective on its own).

You must inform your Western and CAM practitioners of every drug or therapy you're using and report any changes or side effects immediately. Not doing so could result in a potentially dangerous interaction. If you don't tell your practitioners, they can't help you.

Alternative Medical Systems

A medical system encompasses not only the treatments you might receive, but also the philosophy behind the system. In this section, I give you some more detail about the main types of alternative systems that you may encounter while looking to treat your hep C.

Traditional Chinese medicine

What's called traditional Chinese medicine (TCM) began in China and other nearby countries and has been developed over the past 5,000 years. Chinese medicine views each person as a microcosm of the universe. Here are two key principles (among the many) of Chinese medicine:

✔ **Qi:** Also spelled *chi, qi* is life-force energy. You're healthy when your qi is in balance and unhealthy when your qi is out of balance.

✔ **Yin and yang:** Everyone has bits of both yin and yang, which are halves of the same whole. For example, female, night, and wet are considered to be yin, and male, day, and dry are yang. To be in harmony is to have yin and yang balanced within your body.

The purpose of Chinese medicine is to balance your energy channels so that your body, mind, and spirit are in harmony. Chinese medicine provides an excellent way to deal with hepatitis C symptoms and drug-treatment side effects.

Chinese medicine looks at patients as a whole, so diagnoses take into account the season, weather, and other aspects of the environment. If you visit a Chinese-medicine practitioner, he or she will ask questions, listen to your voice and breathing patterns, observe your skin and tongue, feel your pulse, and put the information together for a diagnosis.

Your diagnosis will reflect an energy imbalance in some part of your body. On the basis of this diagnosis, the practitioner may recommend acupuncture, herbs, nutritional counseling, and/or Qigong exercises. Here's a closer look at some of the components of TCM:

✔ **Acupuncture, acupressure, and moxibustion:** Energy travels by invisible channels (meridians) throughout the body; each channel represents a distinct system, such as the liver channel or gallbladder channel. *Acupuncture* is the use of thin needles to stimulate points (gates to open energy flow) on the meridians. *Acupressure* is the stimulation of points with the fingers and can be done at home. *Moxibustion* is the burning of Chinese herbs safely on the body at specific points to warm energy channels.

✔ **Chinese herbs:** Chinese medicine has more than 30 different herb formulations (each containing a complex of individual herbs) for treating different aspects of hepatitis C. For this reason, it's essential to find a TCM practitioner who's an expert at diagnosis and herbal treatment. Some Chinese herbs are actually derived from animal or mineral products — so they're not technically herbs but are used in the same way as herbs.

✔ **Nutrition:** Your practitioner will advise you on what types of foods to include and avoid. Different nutritional strategies are used, depending on your Western and Chinese diagnoses.

✔ **Exercise, breathing, and meditation:** Chinese exercises such as Qigong and T'ai Chi are forms of mind–body treatments that use breathing, movement, and meditation to achieve energy balancing and relaxation. See Chapter 13 for more information.

Within this chapter, I'm able only to scratch the surface of this ancient and vast subject. If you want more info on Chinese medicine and its relation to hepatitis C treatment, Misha Ruth Cohen (a Chinese-medicine practitioner) and Robert Gish (a distinguished liver specialist) have written, with Kalia Doner, *The Hepatitis C Help Book: A Groundbreaking Treatment Program Combining Western and Eastern Medicine for Maximum Wellness and Healing* (St. Martin's Press, 2001).

To find a practitioner, follow the information at the end of this chapter, and consult the Web site for the National Certification Commission for Acupuncture and Oriental Medicine at www. nccaom.org. It has a database of certified practitioners of TCM in the United States and Canada.

Ayurvedic medicine

Ayurvedic medicine has been practiced in India for more than 5,000 years. *Ayurveda* is a system that integrates everything about a person and his surroundings, similar to traditional Chinese medicine. Ayurveda calls the life-force energy *prana*. Prana is concentrated in seven different energy centers in the body, called *chakras.* In ayurveda medicine, you're defined as having a combination of the three *doshas* (energy patterns):

✔ **Vata:** When *vata* predominates, you are vivacious and thin, chill easily, sleep poorly, and have digestive problems.

✔ **Pitta:** If you have a tendency toward *pitta,* you're intense, with a medium build, and prone to liver disorders.

✔ **Kapha:** Folks with lots of *kapha* are graceful, gain weight easily, and are prone to allergies and asthma.

I have space here to provide only a brief generalization. Most people have a combination of each of the doshas, but one or two usually dominate your personality, body type, and health. Depending on your predominant dosha, your treatment will include the following:

✔ Herbs

✔ Nutrition

✔ Lifestyle changes

✔ Detoxification

✔ Yoga

✔ Breathing and meditation

Finding a practitioner is much easier in India than in the United States. The Ayurvedic Institute (www.ayurveda.com) in Albuquerque, New Mexico, is one resource for information.

Herbal medicine

Traditional Chinese medicine and ayurveda both use herbs as part of their medical system. Herbs are used in many parts of the world for healing purposes. Even conventional medicine uses some herbs, after distinct active chemicals have been isolated, tested, and then synthesized.

Treating yourself with herbs for hepatitis C can be dangerous, let alone expensive and ineffective. Thousands of herbs are reported to have different effects on the liver or immune system, and some of those effects can be toxic (see Chapter 12). Only a skilled and knowledgeable practitioner can correctly prescribe the right combination of herbs. Here's how hazardous self-treatment can be: In a book about using herbs for hepatitis C, I found suggestions to use certain herbs that are known to potentially cause liver damage! I recommend visiting a licensed practitioner of Chinese medicine, a naturopathic doctor (see the section "Naturopathy," later in this chapter), or another CAM practitioner who has expertise and experience with hepatitis C.

To make your herbal experience safe and effective:

✔ Consult only an experienced herbal practitioner.

✔ Buy reputable products that are tested for safety and are standardized by the United States Pharmacopeia (www.usp.org).

✔ Look at reviews or endorsements of products:

- American Botanical Council (www.herbalgram.org) gives access (for a price) to German Commission E reports (which is the German equivalent of the U.S. FDA and is the international authority on herbs).

- ConsumerLab.com (www.consumerlab.com) performs its own testing of some herbal or supplement products.

✔ Start with low doses.

✔ Tell your conventional doctor and any other medical practitioners which herbs you're taking.

The next sections provide some general information about herbs that are sometimes used in the treatment of hepatitis C. I'm not advising you to buy them or use them; neither am I providing information on how and when to take them. I'm simply relaying some information. If you want to take these or other herbs, see a qualified practitioner.

Silymarin (Milk thistle)

German research has focused on the silymarin component of the seeds of the milk thistle plant. Silymarin is able to protect the liver from damage. The milk thistle plant is native to the Mediterranean area and grows wild in Europe, California, and Australia.

Schisandra (Wu Wei Zi)

Schisandra is a Chinese herb used to treat hepatitis and poor liver function and also is a general tonic to strengthen the entire body. Schisandra is a woody vine grown in northeast China that produces pink flowers. The berries are used in herbal preparations. The active ingredients in schisandra include chemicals called lignans, triterpenes, oils, and vitamins. Large doses can cause heartburn.

Ginseng (Panax ginseng; Ren Shen)

This most famous of all Chinese herbs is native to parts of China, Russia, and North Korea but is no longer found in the wild. The root of the ginseng plant has been shown to help the body deal with stress, fatigue, and cold.

Homeopathy

A German doctor developed homeopathic science in the late 1700s. *Homeopathy* uses the similar *(homeo)* to cure disease *(pathy)*. Homeopathic remedies are substances that in large doses would give symptoms but are given in minuscule doses believed to heal those same symptoms. The remedies are extremely diluted in water or alcohol in a special way *(potentiation)*. Homeopathic remedies can be used to treat acute symptoms or entire *constitutions* (the general picture of a person that predisposes them to certain illnesses.)

Conventional medicine and scientists have more trouble understanding homeopathy than other CAM therapies because homeopathic medicines are so diluted that probably none of the original substance remains.

For treatment for a chronic illness like hepatitis C, you need to make sure that your homeopath is experienced. The homeopath will ask questions about your general health to determine the right remedy for you. Some MDs, DOs, chiropractors, and naturopathic physicians (NPs) practice homeopathy, so you may be covered by your insurance.

For more information on homeopathy or to find a practitioner, consult the National Center for Homeopathy (www.homeopathic. org) or the American Institute of Homeopathy (www.homeopathy usa.org).

Naturopathy

Naturopathy is medicine with a holistic twist. A naturopathic physician or naturopathic doctor (ND) is trained in Western medicine, similar to the training that an MD receives, but with extra training in nutrition (food and vitamin therapy), herbal medicine, Chinese medicine, and homeopathy, among other treatments. Some health insurance covers visits to naturopathic physicians. To find a naturopathic physician, contact the American Association of Naturopathic Physicians (www.naturopathic.org).

Finding Complementary and Alternative Providers

To find a CAM practitioner, you can consult the following sources:

- ✔ Your primary care physician or liver specialist
- ✔ Professional CAM associations (see the specific CAM treatment sections, earlier in this chapter)
- ✔ State licensing or regulatory associations
- ✔ Other CAM providers
- ✔ Schools of alternative care
- ✔ Hepatitis C support groups

Just as you have questions and requirements of your conventional medical doctors, you must question your CAM practitioners. Ask a new practitioner these questions:

- ✔ What is your qualification for this particular health practice?
- ✔ Do you accept my insurance? What are your charges?
- ✔ How long have you been treating people with hepatitis C?
- ✔ How many people do you treat a year with hepatitis C?

Make sure that the CAM practitioner is open to your opinions of conventional medicine, especially if you hope to combine treatments.

Part III
Living a Good Life with Hep C

The 5th Wave
By Rich Tennant

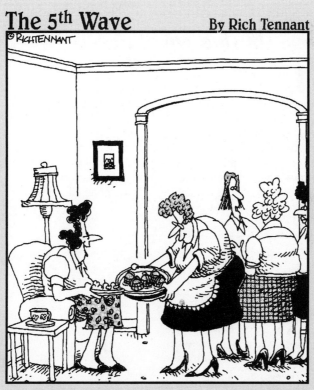

"Oh, no thank you, Bernice. My doctor's told me to avoid foods containing too much iron, pesticides, or hand grenades."

In this part . . .

*H*epatitis C is a chronic illness that can last for decades. In this part, I describe how to help manage your hep C and stay strong and calm. You can keep your body and mind healthy by eating well, avoiding toxic substances, exercising, relaxing, and getting emotional support. I include information to help you deal with the practical issues of disclosing your hepatitis C to others and dealing with changes in your work or financial situation. I also explain how having a positive attitude goes a long way toward feeling better.

Chapter 11

Eating and Drinking for Health

● ●

In This Chapter

▶ Examining the hepatitis C needs for good nutrition

▶ Defining digestion

▶ Getting a balanced diet

▶ Dealing with hep C symptoms

▶ Choosing healthy meals in restaurants

▶ Selecting the right beverages

▶ Making meal plans

▶ Dealing with cirrhosis

▶ Maintaining a healthy weight

● ●

*W*hen you're living with a chronic illness like hepatitis C, healthy eating can make a big difference in your symptoms and mood. Making healthy choices by avoiding certain foods and eating others may help protect you from further liver damage or cancer. You're in charge when it comes to your diet. In this chapter, I provide general information that uses common sense to design a healthy eating style. You may not be able to follow all the suggestions, but even small changes are helpful.

Everyone is different in age, gender, genetics, length of illness, general health, liver condition, food preferences, and symptoms that interfere with eating. So, I'm giving general nutritional information for the average adult. I'm not recommending any supplements in this chapter. For advice that's specific to your condition and situation, visit your doctor or a qualified nutritionist.

If you wish to delve further into nutrition charts, calories, or levels of specific nutrients, consult a nutrition book. *Nutrition For Dummies*, 3rd edition, by Carol Ann Rinzler (published by Wiley), is an excellent

source of more detailed information. Also, Health Canada has published "Hepatitis C: Nutrition Care Canadian Guidelines for Health
Care Providers" on its Web site (`www.phac-aspc.gc.ca/hepc/
hepatitis_c/pdf/nutritionCareGuidelines`).

Why Nutrition Matters with Hepatitis C

Nutrition matters — right down to the smallest level in your body.
Each cell is made of the byproducts of food that you've eaten in
the past. No, you can't take a few cells, put them under the microscope, and spot that toasted cheese sandwich with fries. Not
exactly. Seeing the effects of what you eat on a cellular level isn't
easy, even for scientists. So take a look at the effects of food on a
larger level. Have you ever noticed that

- ✔ If you eat too much or too little, you gain or lose a few pounds?

- ✔ If you drink too much, you feel hung over? (I hope those days
  are all in your past, because alcohol is off limits when you
  have hep C; see Chapter 12.)

- ✔ If you eat too much chocolate, you get a headache or nausea?

- ✔ If you've ever been really hungry or headachy and then eaten
  a good meal, you feel wonderful?

If you can answer yes to any of these questions, you have some reference for noticing that what you eat really affects your body and
your mood.

Good nutrition is key to getting well when you have hepatitis C.
The cells of your immune system (which fight the hepatitis C
virus) and the cells of your liver depend on what you eat to do
their job. Eating the right foods and avoiding the wrong ones can
also help you with the symptoms of hep C and side effects of medication. Here's some important nutritional advice:

- ✔ Drink enough water.

- ✔ Don't drink alcohol.

- ✔ Avoid chemical additives and pesticides in your food.

- ✔ Eat regularly throughout the day.

- ✔ Eat a balanced diet that contains the three major food groups:
  carbohydrates, fat, and protein.

✔ Eat a wide variety and quantity of fruits, vegetables, and grains (preferably organic) to get phytochemicals, vitamins, and minerals

✔ Take supplements as recommended by your healthcare provider.

✔ Avoid or limit caffeine, junk food, processed food, fried food, and high-sugar food.

The rest of this chapter elaborates on these suggestions and addresses specific issues that apply when you have hepatitis C and symptoms.

Connecting the Pieces of the Digestion Puzzle

Before getting into the nutrition nitty-gritty, you need to understand where food goes and what it does when it gets into the body. *Digestion* is the process of breaking down food into energy and nutrients (see Figure 11-1 for an outline of the digestive system).

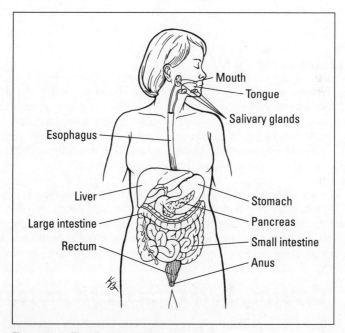

Figure 11-1: The digestive system.

Digestion begins with the first spoonful of delicious food:

1. The saliva in your mouth contains enzymes that start breaking food down, and your teeth tear the food. The tongue pushes the food down toward the esophagus.

2. The food, wet with saliva, is pumped through the esophagus to the stomach.

3. The stomach uses acidic gastric juice along with a pumping action to break down food into a paste.

4. The digested food paste is sent to the small intestine, which is many feet long and rolled up inside your lower abdomen.

5. Carbohydrates, proteins, and fats are absorbed into the bloodstream, and the waste is sent to the large intestine (also called the colon) for elimination as feces from the rectum.

The pancreas, liver, and gallbladder don't physically break down the actual food, but they help process nutrients into a form that can be used by individual cells of the body. The liver, in particular, filters any out toxic chemicals (such as pesticides) or drugs (such as antibiotics) present in food, stores sugar (as glycogen), processes fats and cholesterol, and makes bile. (For more info on the role of the liver in digestion and its other key functions, see Chapter 4.)

Balancing Your Diet

The more you vary the types of foods you eat within the different food groups, the better chance you have of giving your body the nutrition it needs. A balanced diet consists of appropriate amounts of the three basic nutrients — carbs, fats, and protein — along with attention paid to the vitamins, minerals, and phytochemicals (a relatively new player in the nutrition game).

In the following sections, I provide a basic rundown of these nutrients, a brief summary of their function, and foods that have them. You'll notice a plant theme developing, so I'll warn you upfront: Don't be surprised if you run out to get colorful fruits and veggies and some yummy whole-grains after reading these sections!

Covering carbs, fats, and protein

If you've read Chapter 2, you may notice that the following nutrients are the same chemical substances that you find in cells.

✔ **Carbohydrates** give you energy. They make up the majority of a healthy diet. Aim to get 45 to 65 percent of your calories from carbohydrates. *Complex carbohydrates,* which are found in foods like potatoes, pasta, and rice, also contain vitamins and fiber. *Dietary fiber's* role in the body is different from that of other carbs — it aids digestion instead of providing energy.

✔ **Fats** are essential to provide energy, to make certain vitamins, and to help the body stay warm. Aim to get 20 to 35 percent of your calories from fat.

Cholesterol, a type of fat, is made by the liver (see Chapter 4) but is also found in certain foods. Table 11-1 contains a breakdown of the different types of fat. In general, avoid the fats that are solid at room temperature: saturated fats, trans fats, and cholesterol. Liquid oils are a better way to fulfill the body's need for fats.

✔ **Protein** is essential for cell growth and repair and for production of hormones, antibodies, and enzymes. Aim for 10 to 30–35 percent of your calories to come from protein.

Proteins are made up of amino acids. Some nine amino acids are called *essential* because the body can't make them on its own. A protein that has all the essential amino acids is called a *complete protein.* All animal-based foods, including eggs and dairy products, are complete proteins.

If you don't eat any animal-derived food (vegan), you should know that soybeans, spinach, and quinoa (a grain) are complete plant-based proteins. Other protein sources, like beans, rice, and corn, are incomplete. The key is to combine foods with incomplete proteins to get all the amino acids you need, like eating rice along with beans.

Table 11-1	Description of Fats in Food
Type of Fat or Cholesterol	*Source*
Saturated fatty acid	Animal products: Meat, dairy products, coconut oil, and palm oil.
Dietary cholesterol	Animal products: Eggs, beef, fish, and dairy products.
Trans fatty acid	Processed (hydrogenated) forms of vegetable oils found in margarine or shortening. Found in many processed foods and fried foods.
Monounsaturated fatty acid	Vegetable oils: Canola, olive, and peanut.
Polyunsaturated fatty acid	Vegetable oils: Safflower, sunflower, corn, flaxseed, and canola. Also in seafood.

Carbohydrates, fats, and protein all provide calories and are all essential for health. A balanced diet is one in which your meals and snacks contain protein, fats, and carbohydrates, or at least protein and carbohydrates. When including fats, add the healthy fats from vegetables and fish.

See Figure 11-2 for guidelines for a balanced diet that I adapted from the U.S. Department of Agriculture and Department of Health and Human Services recommendations for healthy eating (www.health.gov/dietaryguidelines). In these days of super-sizing, figuring out what a serving size is can be confusing, so I added the basic amounts of a serving for each major food group.

Don't eat raw shellfish when you have hep C because they could contain hepatitis A or other viruses or bacteria. Raw mollusks like uncooked clams or oysters can be infected with the bacteria *Vibrio vulnificus,* which could be dangerous when you have liver disease.

Don't try any diet that limits one of the basic food groups (such as carbohydrates, protein, or fat) unless specifically under medical supervision of someone who knows your hep C status. Each of the food groups is essential for good health.

Viewing vitamins and minerals

Vitamins are essential for body function. Table 11-2 explains how they keep you healthy and where to find them.

Don't take any supplement without the advice of your healthcare practitioner. In this chapter, I'm advising you on how to get nutri-ents from your food. If you still need supplementation, your doctor can properly advise you.

Table 11-2	Benefits and Sources of Vitamins	
Vitamin	*What It Does*	*Where to Find It*
Vitamin A (beta carotene)	Supports mucous membranes, immune system,adrenals, and eyes.	Yellow and orange fruits and vegetables (such as carrots, apricots, mangoes, and yams), and green leafy vegetables.
Vitamin D	Supports bone, teeth, and muscles.	Sunshine is the best source. Also fish, eggs, and dairy products.

Vitamin	What It Does	Where to Find It
Vitamin E	Helps tissue healing, cell structure. Protects against oxidation (*antioxidant*, thought to protect against tissue damage and aging).	Wheat germ, egg yolks, vegetable oils, nuts, seeds, green eafy vegetables, land avocados.
Vitamin K	Helps with blood clotting and bone formation.	Dark green, leafy vegetables.
Vitamin B1 (thiamin)	Works in carbohydrate metabolism, giving you energy.	Whole grains, fruits, vegetables, seeds, and meat.
Vitamin B2 (riboflavin)	Essential for digesting proteins and carbohydrates.	Meat, fish, poultry, eggs, milk, whole wheat, dairy, and dark green vegetables.
Vitamin B3 (niacin)	Important for nervous system functioning.	Poultry, dairy, eggs, and whole grains.
Vitamin B6 (pyridoxine)	Helps with breakdown of proteins, carbohydrates, and fats.	Poultry, fish, soybeans, and potatoes.
Vitamin B12 (cobalamin)	Keeps red blood cells healthy.	Meat, fish, poultry, eggs, and dairy products. Note that this isn't made by plants, so vegetarians who don't eat animal products should eat products that have vitamin B12 added or speak to their doctor about supplements.
Biotin	Helps in metabolism of fatty acids and carbohydrates.	Egg yolk, yeast, nuts, and beans.
Folic acid (a B vitamin)	Helps in cell and tissue growth.	Beans and dark green, leafy vegetables.
Vitamin C	Important for wound healing and immune response. Like vitamin E, vitamin C is an antioxidant.	Fruits and vegetables, especially rose hips, red peppers, broccoli, kale, citrus fruits, and strawberries.

Food	Examples	Serving Size	Number of Servings/Day
Dairy Products	Milk, cheese, yogurt (Low fat is preferable)	1 cup of milk is equal to 1 cup yogurt, 1 1/2 – 2 ounces of cheese	3 cups milk
Meat and beans	Beef, lamb, pork	1 ounce equivalent is 1 ounce lean meat, poultry, or fish; 1 egg; 1/4 cup cooked dry beans or tofu; 1 tablespoon peanut butter; 1/2 ounce nuts or seeds	5 1/2 ounce equivalents
Fish and seafood	Salmon, shrimp		
Poultry	Chicken, turkey		
Legumes	Soybeans, peas, beans, peanuts		
Grains	Bread, cereal, pasta, rice (Half or more should come from whole grains)	1 ounce (1 serving) of grains is 1/2 cup cooked rice, pasta, or cereal; 1 ounce dry pasta or rice; 1 slice bread; 1 small muffin; 1 cup ready-to-eat cereal flakes	6 ounces
Fruit	Apple, banana, orange, nectarine, grapes	1 cup or 2 servings is equivalent to 1 cup raw or cooked fruit, 1 cup juice	2 cups or 4 servings
Vegetables	Beans spinach, broccoli, squash, carrot, pepper	1 cup or 2 servings is equivalent to 2 cups leafy salad greens, 1 cup cooked veggies, 1 cup vegetable juice	2.5 cups or 5 servings

Figure 11-2: The amounts shown are based on a 2,000-calories-per-day diet. You may need a little more or less, depending on your calorie intake.

Minerals also play an essential role in body function. They can be called *major* or *trace,* depending on how much is normally found in the body. Minerals come from rocks and metal ores, which plants pick up from the soil and animals pick up from plants. When you eat plants or animals, you're getting the minerals into your body.

Sounding off about sodium

Keeping your salt or sodium intake down is a good idea. Salt is another name for sodium chloride, and if you eat foods with sodium, that's the same as salt to your body. For people without cirrhosis, keep your sodium levels at 2.4 grams (2,400 milligrams) per day, which is the recommended daily amount. If you have cirrhosis or ascites (see Chapter 4), follow your doctor's advice about salt intake. Here are some ways to monitor your sodium use:

✔ Stop using the saltshaker and use lemon juice, herbs, and spices instead.

✔ Read nutrition labels to check the levels of sodium in your foods.

✔ Watch for these substances: monosodium glutamate (a flavor enhancer found in many snack foods and Chinese meals), sodium benzoate and sodium nitrate (which keep foods from spoiling), sodium caseinate (a food thickener), sodium citrate (which keeps the carbonation going in sodas), and sodium saccharin (a sweetener without calories but with the sodium).

✔ Watch for sodium in over-the-counter products in the form of sodium ascorbate (a form of vitamin C), sodium bicarbonate, and sodium citrate (used as antacids).

Major minerals include the following.

✔ **Calcium** is important for bones and teeth. Find calcium in green vegetables and in dairy and soy products.

✔ **Magnesium** plays a role in energy production and nerve function. Find magnesium in soybeans, whole grains, fish, nuts, bananas, dairy products, and green vegetables.

✔ **Phosphorus** helps in bone and teeth formation, as well as in energy metabolism in the body. Eat fish, poultry, eggs, and whole grains to get your phosphorus.

✔ **Potassium** helps the nervous system, heart, and muscles. Eat fruit, potatoes, and yogurt to get enough potassium.

✔ **Sodium** plays a role in regulating and balancing fluid levels in the body. Most foods and water contain salt. Sodium is especially high in salted foods, soy sauce, cheese, and seafood. See the "Sounding off about sodium" sidebar in this chapter for more information.

The trace minerals needed by the body are boron, chromium, cobalt, copper, iodine, iron, manganese, selenium, silicon, sulfur, and zinc. These three trace elements are of special interest with hep C:

✔ **Selenium** works with vitamin E as an antioxidant, which may help heal tissue damage from hepatitis C. Find it in seafood, meat, eggs, dairy products, vegetables, and grains.

✔ **Zinc** aids the nervous system and boosts the immune systems — two parts of the body that take a hit from hep C infection. Find zinc in brewer's yeast, seafood, whole grains, nuts, seeds, and vegetables.

✔ **Iron** is important to maintain energy levels. High levels are found in liver and red meat, egg yolks, wheat germ, and oysters. Whole grains, fish, vegetables, and raisins are other sources.

Your doctor will monitor your blood for levels of iron. Too much iron in your blood can harm your liver (which stores iron). Your doctor may tell you to take a vitamin supplement without iron.

Focusing on phytochemicals

Phytochemicals are an amazing array of medicinal chemicals made only by plants. Different phytochemicals are found in fruits, vegetables, beans, and grains. As herbal practitioners and pharmaceutical companies alike study plants for their healing properties, thousands of different phytochemicals have been identified and more will be revealed about their health-boosting ability, including cancer prevention.

Fitting fruits and veggies into your diet

Here are some ways to get more fruits and veggies in your diet. Think color, variety, and freshness when going for plant nutrition.

✔ Keep some veggies cut up and ready to go.

✔ Always have some ready-to-eat fruit on hand, such as apples, oranges, grapes, or berries.

✔ Keep some frozen fruit in the freezer to add to yogurt or smoothies.

✔ Make vegetable soup with a variety of vegetables.

✔ Drink 100 percent fruit or vegetable juice instead of soda.

✔ Use lettuce leaves to top a sandwich.

✔ Make sure to have a fruit or vegetable, or both, with every meal or snack.

✔ Try making stir-fried vegetables. Serve with rice or pasta.

Each plant has different phytochemicals in different amounts and combinations. If you eat a plant-based food, you get this phytochemical "brew." When you buy an isolated phytochemical in pill form, no one really has determined whether you get the same benefit.

Go for color! Eat a wide variety of fruits and vegetables daily from different plant families and different colors so that you can give yourself a wide array of phytochemicals, vitamins, and minerals.

Some of the phytochemicals, their properties, and food sources include the following:

✔ **Carotenoids:** Carotenoids have powerful antioxidant properties, which can slow cell damage (including inflammation) and prevent cancer. They're found in yellow and dark green fruits and vegetables and in tomatoes. (You may have heard of the carotenoid in tomatoes: lycopene.)

✔ **Flavonoids:** Flavonoids are also antioxidants. Celery, cranberries, onions, kale, broccoli, apples, cherries, berries, green and black tea, purple grape juice, parsley, soybeans, tomatoes, eggplant, and thyme are ways to get more flavonoids.

✔ **Phytoestrogens:** They have activities similar to the female hormone estrogen. These are antioxidants and may inhibit cancer and bone loss and improve cholesterol. One type, *isoflavones,* is found in soybeans and soy products. Another type, *lignans,* is found in the fiber layer of whole grains (such as rice and wheat), berries, and some seeds and vegetables.

✔ **Isothiocyanates:** These sulfur-containing compounds help reduce the risk of cancer. Cruciferous vegetables like cabbage, broccoli, Brussels sprouts, cauliflower, and kale have isothiocyanates. These vegetables can give off a smelly aroma when they're cooked, so try them raw or cold if the smell disturbs you.

Do you like your food spicy or highly flavored? The *capsaicin* found in hot red peppers helps reduce inflammation and pain. And if you eat fresh garlic, onion, chives, and leeks, you'll get the phytochemical called *allicin,* which may have antibiotic and antiviral properties.

Practicing moderation

Good nutrition isn't just knowing what to eat but also what *not* to eat. The foods and drinks to have in moderation include the following:

✔ **Junk foods and fast foods:** Monitor your consumption of those salty, crunchy snacks and temptations that satisfy your sweet tooth. This chapter is filled with suggestions for trying fruits (instead of sweets) and vegetables and grains (instead of salty fried foods).

✔ **Caffeine:** Coffee, tea, chocolate, and many soft drinks contain caffeine. Limit them to two to three servings a day or fewer. Try decaffeinated drinks like seltzer, decaffeinated coffee and tea, juice, or water instead of caffeine.

✔ **Fats and oils:** This category includes salad dressing, cooking oil, butter, and sour cream. For cooking and baking, use oils like olive or canola instead of butter or margarine (refer to Table 11-1). Avoid fatty meats and fats from processed foods, cakes, pastries, chips, and fried foods because these fats are more likely to be saturated or trans fatty acids and may contribute to digestive problems (like nausea and indigestion). The bad fats also increase the "bad" LDL cholesterol.

Try tweaking some of your favorite treats to make them healthier:

✔ If you love French fries, try eating baked or grilled potatoes.

✔ If you love chocolate, eat tiny amounts of only very good-quality chocolate.

✔ If you love iced desserts, get an ice cream maker and put in your own organic ingredients.

✔ If you love cookies, try oatmeal and whole-wheat cookies.

If you have special occasions when you must have steak and cake or if you just have a love for French fries that won't die, balance your other meals that day and the next by including lots of fresh veggies and fruit, drinking lots of water, and reducing your intake of fat and sodium.

Enjoying food

Just because you're eating healthy meals doesn't mean that you can't get some pleasure from food! Don't forgo enjoyment of your food. You can find satisfaction by trying mindful eating:

✔ Pay attention to what you're eating.

✔ Chew slowly.

✔ Give thanks for your food.

✔ Eat in a calm environment.

Creating healthy meals or snacks

Here are some ideas for healthy snacks or small meals. Keep some of these items around so you don't run out of food when you need it and then have to grab something quick and less healthy:

✔ Lowfat yogurt mixed with fruit or nuts

✔ Crackers with lowfat cream cheese and cucumber

✔ Whole-wheat toast spread with nut butters (such as almond, peanut, or sesame seed butter) and apple slices

✔ Sliced veggies served with lowfat yogurt or low-salt bean dip and salsa

✔ Vegetable bean soup with crusty whole-wheat bread

✔ Hard-boiled eggs sliced into a spinach salad

✔ Lowfat cheese with slices of pear

✔ Vegetable bean chili with brown rice

✔ Turkey slices with coleslaw

✔ Fresh or frozen fruit smoothies with yogurt and juice

✔ Trail mix made of a dried fruit and nut combination

Another tip is to treat yourself to foods that soothe. Try foods that are nourishing and a treat for the senses, such as crunchy tart apples, sweet cold watermelon slices, and thick yogurt with banana slices. Or make the comfort foods that remind you of your childhood. For example, you may like hot foods such as vegetable or chicken soup or cups of milky tea. Hot cereals are also comforting. At holiday times, eat small portions of ceremonial or special foods.

Easing Hep C Symptoms

Some symptoms of hep C make it difficult to eat. You may have nausea, vomiting, diarrhea, or no appetite for food at all. Follow these tips to deal with these side effects of hep C or interferon treatment:

✔ **Keep a daily food journal.** Monitor your diet so you can learn which foods trigger your symptoms. Recording the foods you eat helps you make sure that your diet is balanced and you're getting enough calories.

✔ **Identify any trigger foods that make you nauseated.** This is another use for your food journal. Identify these trigger foods and then avoid them. If the smell of food makes you queasy, eat food that is cool or at room temperature, use indoor fans, or cook food outdoors.

✔ **Avoid greasy or fatty foods.** Fatty, greasy food doesn't sit well in the stomach and can contribute to indigestion.

✔ **Eat small, healthy meals regularly throughout the day, even when you're not very hungry.** To maintain your energy and keep your body functioning throughout the day, eat your meals at regular intervals. You may want to eat lots of smaller meals every three to four hours or the three square meals of breakfast, lunch, and dinner. Small meals are easier to eat if you're not hungry, and they'll help ward off fatigue.

If you are having trouble eating, get full quickly, or don't have much of an appetite, try these suggestions:

✔ Drink water or juice at nonmeal times. If you drink liquid at mealtime, it may fill you up quickly, and you won't eat enough.

✔ Drink juice, milk, or milkshakes instead of low-calorie fluids like tea, broth, or coffee. To try to get more nutrition from everything you put in your mouth, have drinks that provide you with some nourishment.

✔ Make sure to eat when your appetite is best. Get some nourishment in your system when you can.

✔ Try eating different-tasting foods — perhaps something bitter, sweet, salty, or sour — to stimulate your appetite.

✔ If you have diarrhea or vomiting, drink more fluids.

✔ Talk to your doctor about taking zinc supplements, which might improve the taste of foods.

Going Out to Eat

You've probably noticed that restaurant portions have expanded over the years, which is often called the "supersizing" phenomenon. And despite the popularity of fad diets and greater emphasis on healthy options, much restaurant food is still high in fat, sugar, and calories. You can, however, make your restaurant experience healthier and more enjoyable (what's to enjoy if you feel ill after your restaurant experience?).

Sometimes, you just can't avoid eating in a fast-food restaurant: You're rushing around running errands all day, you're traveling on business and in a hurry, or you have to find a place with food your kids will actually eat. Here are some suggestions for eating healthier even in a fast-food place:

- ✔ Choose a salad (but go for the lowfat dressing), yogurt and fruit, grilled chicken, or a baked potato.

- ✔ Skip the sauces, mayonnaise, and heavy dressings. Try mustard instead.

- ✔ Omit the cheese from your burgers or nachos.

- ✔ Avoid fried chicken and chicken nuggets.

- ✔ Order a small single burger rather than the large one.

- ✔ If you must have fries, go with a small order rather than large.

If you're going to a sit-down restaurant, try to plan in advance what type of food will be good for you that day. Try these tips to keep your meal healthy:

- ✔ Ask for all salad dressings and sauces on the side.

- ✔ Order soups that aren't cream-based.

- ✔ Skip the bread or avoid the butter.

- ✔ Split an entrée with someone else.

- ✔ Take some food home.

- ✔ Try eating an appetizer as your main course.

- ✔ Order your meat or fish baked, broiled, or dry-sautéed.

- ✔ Tell your server what your needs are.

- ✔ Order steamed vegetables.

- ✔ Choose fruit, sorbet, or other nonfat items for dessert.

Drinking Like a King

Nutrition includes not only solid food but also the liquids you put in a glass. The basic instructions for a person with hep C can be summed up simply: Drink lots of water and skip the alcohol.

Getting your eight glasses of water

Drinking water is essential to managing hep C or interferon treatment side effects. Consider these watery facts:

- ✔ A healthy person can live for around 40 days without food but can go only 7 or fewer days without water.

- ✔ Water is the main constituent of your body (about two-thirds water).

- ✔ Water flushes toxins out of your body.

The eight glasses of water a day is actually an estimate. You may need more or less, depending on your size and activity level. What type of water do you drink now? Here's a rundown of different types of water:

- ✔ **Tap water:** It probably contains chlorine (purifier) or fluoride (to prevent tooth decay). Water from the tap may have a taste of certain minerals and may contain some pollutants or toxins. Contact your local water department or health department to get more advice. You can always get your water tested.

- ✔ **Filtered water:** Different filtration systems are available. Read the information to see which microorganisms and chemicals the filter keeps out of your water.

- ✔ **Distilled water:** This water is boiled, and the steam is caught and cooled. Because there are no minerals, this water has little taste.

- ✔ **Bottled water:** The quality and taste of the water depend on the original source (spring or public water supply) and method of treatment (like reverse osmosis, carbon filtration, or microfiltration) before bottling. Read the labels carefully, though you may not get much information.

Which water is best? Do your homework and compare information on bottled water and any filtration system you use in your home. Get the best filtration system or bottled water you can afford.

People generally stand in one of two camps: "Tap water is perfectly fine for me" or "I won't drink anything but bottled water." Whichever water you choose to drink, just drink it throughout the day and don't let yourself get thirsty.

 If you want to do homework on your tap or well water, check out the U.S. Environmental Protection Agency's safe-water Web site (www.epa.gov/safewater). *Consumer Reports* also has information on bottled water, which you can see on its Web site (www.consumer reports.org) or find at your local library.

 If you use purified water, make sure to use it for ice cubes; cooking (especially rice and grains, which absorb water); reconstituting juices; and all your drinks, including tea, coffee, and smoothies.

Drinking socially without alcohol

 You're following your doctor's orders, and you've stopped drinking alcoholic beverages. Now what do you drink instead? In a restaurant, club, or bar — or when you're hanging out with friends at home — try one of these nonalcoholic beverages:

- ✔ Club soda on ice with a twist of lemon or lime

- ✔ A frozen drink mix without the alcohol

- ✔ Hot or iced teas (but not ones that have too much caffeine or dangerous herbs, which you can read about in Chapter 12)

- ✔ Orange, apple, tomato, cranberry, or pineapple juice

- ✔ Water, sparkling or flat, on ice or straight up, with or without lemon

- ✔ Regular and diet sodas

- ✔ Sparkly ginger ale (ideal when everyone else is drinking champagne)

- ✔ Grape juice (red or white) instead of wine (red or white)

Planning Your Meals

When you plan ahead, you can save yourself stress and confusion. Be realistic about what you need, what you can afford, and what's within your ability to prepare. Depending on where you live and/or your financial situation, some foods (such as organic produce) may not be easy to get.

If you want to change to a healthy eating style, make changes gradually by eliminating the dangerous foods or drinks first. Then add some healthy choices.

Using a food diary

Some healthcare professionals may ask you to keep a food diary or journal. This tool is valuable, especially when you're having symptoms from hep C or interferon treatment. Try to write down everything you eat at meals and in between.

You can keep this information in your hep C notebook. Create a list from this chapter of new foods to try (like broccoli or lowfat yogurt) and another list of foods to work on eliminating or reducing (like potato chips or ice cream).

Shopping smartly

Preparing food is a big job: Ask any chef or mom or dad with kids to feed. With hep C, you may have the additional challenges of a limited budget, limited energy, nausea, or even aversion to specific foods.

Here are some tips to help you be a smart shopper:

✔ Make a food budget.

✔ Plan meals in advance.

✔ Use a shopping list.

✔ Don't shop for food on an empty stomach (because junk food becomes too tempting).

Experts in organization recommend using preprinted lists each time you shop. When you have figured out what works for you, based on your budget, symptoms, and taste buds, create your own customized lists:

✔ Foods to always have on hand in the house

✔ Foods to buy weekly and monthly

✔ Foods to buy every few days

Being organized takes away the stress of being unorganized.

Use a friend or delivery service to get food in an emergency, but keep food in the house for when you're not well enough to go shopping. Here are some suggestions for foods to have on hand:

✔ **In the freezer:** Sliced bread, frozen veggies, and soup

✔ **In the cupboard:** Beans, tuna, rice, pasta, healthy soup, applesauce, and potatoes

✔ **In the fridge:** Apples, carrots, peanut butter, yogurt, eggs, and juice

Reading labels

When selecting packaged foods to buy or eat, you see all kinds of information on the labels. Front labels may say that the food is "natural," "lowfat" or "low sodium." This part of the label is more advertisement than real information. Take a look, but then turn your attention to the real info:

✔ **Nutrition Facts label:** This information is located on the back or side of food products. The "% Daily Value" information (given for a 2,000-calorie diet) can be used as a rough guide of whether a food has high, medium, or low levels of a particular nutrient (check out the "Balancing Your Diet" section, earlier in the chapter).

✔ **List of ingredients:** Check out this info, usually in small print, to see just what goes into the product.

Taking just a bit of time to look at this info can help you be a more educated consumer and make better choices at the supermarket.

Questioning additives and pesticides

Look at a list of ingredients on any box or can in your cupboard. In addition to the foods you'd expect to see, like water or wheat or corn oil, you'll likely find substances (some pronounceable, others not) that serve as colors, flavors, preservatives, or agents to improve food texture (such as emulsifiers and thickeners). Some foods, like bread and orange juice, also have added nutrients (vitamins and minerals).

The U.S. Food and Drug Administration (FDA) regulates the use of additives in foods and requires that they be listed on the label. Food additives surely have their benefits. They can give you extra nutrition (but beware if you're avoiding extra iron), prolong the food's shelf life, and make the product seem more appealing.

 But because all chemicals in food pass through your liver and you probably should avoid taxing your liver (especially if you have cirrhosis), avoiding extra additives is the best solution. If you read labels carefully, you can find products in health stores and even supermarkets that have fewer additives. I'm a realist, though. Unless you're a committed organic macrobiotic farmer, avoiding some additives is nearly impossible. So my suggestion is to avoid extra chemicals — when you can.

What about pesticides? *Pesticides* is a general term for chemicals that are applied to crops to protect them from insects, as well as to keep out weeds (herbicides). Most commercial food is grown with pesticides. Because farm animals eat plants grown with pesticides, these chemicals are also present in dairy and meat products. If you're trying to avoid exposure to pesticides, here are some tips:

- ✔ Eat organic foods (see the next section, "Going organic").
- ✔ Wash your fruits and vegetables carefully with special detergents (available in supermarkets) or water and vinegar.
- ✔ Remove the outer layer of cabbage and lettuce leaves.
- ✔ Scrub and peel all root vegetables, such as carrots and potatoes. Also peel (or give a good scrubbing to) all foods that are waxed, including apples, cucumbers, eggplant, peppers, citrus fruits, and tomatoes. Many fruits and veggies are waxed to make them look good and last longer in the market. The wax may not hurt you, but it can seal in pesticides.

Going organic

Organic food differs from conventionally produced food in the way it is grown, handled, and processed. According to the U.S. Department of Agriculture's National Organic Program information for consumers, organic food isn't prepared with growth hormones, antibiotics, conventional pesticides, or fertilizer from synthetic chemicals or sewage sludge. Check out the Web site for the National Organic Program at www.ams.usda.gov/nop for more information.

Folks choose to have some or all of their food come from organic sources to preserve their health and preserve the environment.

Organic farming is becoming increasingly popular as more people want foods that don't have potentially dangerous chemicals. Organic farming is also thought to have less of a negative impact on the environment. Think about it: Where do the pesticides from farm areas wash off? Into the water supply.

Two problems with obtaining organic foods are availability and cost. The reason conventional farming uses pesticides is that it's cost effective and allows prices to be kept low. If you want to try organic food, here are a few ways to find it:

- ✔ Check out a local health food store.

- ✔ Talk to organic farmers in your area to see whether they provide in-season vegetables locally. Or look for a farmers' market that features organic foods.

- ✔ Grow your own vegetables.

But organic (and all-natural) foods are finding a place in more and more produce sections of local and regional grocery stores. Ask your grocer for help locating these products.

Being aware of the food you eat is what's really important. Whether you choose to eat organic foods or not is your personal decision. To find out more about avoiding exposure to toxic chemicals, see Chapter 12.

Eating Well with Cirrhosis

When you have cirrhosis, paying close attention to your diet is especially important, as is avoiding alcohol (see Chapter 12).

Get specific nutritional guidelines from your doctor, who may refer you to a nutritionist or dietitian. Your doctor may recommend that you do the following:

- ✔ Reduce salt/sodium and fluid (water) intake to avoid ascites or edema complications.

- ✔ Reduce your protein levels or change to vegetable protein to manage a condition that can occur with cirrhosis called encephalopathy (see Chapter 4).

- ✔ Eat more protein if you're malnourished. This situation is an example of why you must get proper medical advice to know whether you should increase or reduce your protein levels.

- ✔ Take supplements to aid your diet. Depending on your liver's level of malfunction, you may not be getting adequate nutrition.

Moving Toward a Healthy Weight

Being overweight can put you at risk of the liver disease called nonalcoholic fatty liver disease (NAFLD). Although you may not have symptoms of NAFLD, it can show up as abnormalities in your liver tests (see Chapter 7) and be clearly defined by a liver biopsy. NAFLD can make your hepatitis C disease worse and lessen your response to interferon drug treatment for hep C (see Chapter 8). Recent stats show that an estimated 65 percent of U.S. adults are overweight or obese.

Being overweight may not be your problem, however. You may be underweight as a result of poor nutrition or difficulty eating because of your hepatitis C.

 To see where you stand on weight issues, calculate your body mass index (BMI). Use your BMI value to determine where your weight is on the scale from underweight to overweight. Use this formula, using pounds and inches:

(Your weight ÷ Your height^2) × 703

The National Heart, Lung, and Blood Institute has a BMI calculator and guidelines on its Web site (www.nhlbisupport.com/bmi). All you have to do is plug in your weight and height.

BMI values from 18.5 to 24.9 are considered to be normal weight. If your BMI is below 18.5, you're underweight. If your BMI is over 24.9, you're overweight. Any value 30 or over is considered obese.

Remember to see your doctor to discuss any concerns about your weight and develop a plan to be healthier.

Losing weight the smart way

Trying to lose weight is a challenge for many people. Supermarket shelves, billboards, and televisions entice us with unhealthy products. You can drive hardly anywhere in the United States without encountering easy access to fast food, coffee, doughnuts, and French fries.

Losing weight is a simple concept: Eat fewer calories than the amount of calories you burn through activity. I'm not going to advocate any diet. But I will tell you to follow common sense, consult your doctor about your weight-loss plan, and take it slowly but surely. Here are suggestions to help you lose weight sensibly:

- ✔ Do some form of exercise three to five times a week (see Chapter 13).

- ✔ Avoid junk food.

- ✔ Avoid fast food.

- ✔ Avoid sugary foods, such as soda, cake, candy, ice cream, and cookies.

- ✔ Avoid fatty foods, such as French fries, fried foods, cream sauces, cheeses, and doughnuts.

- ✔ Eat healthy meals, which I discuss in the section "Balancing Your Diet," earlier in this chapter.

- ✔ To satisfy cravings, keep a supply of cut-up vegetables and fruit in the fridge.

- ✔ Try having bread or potatoes without butter, coffee without sugar, lowfat yogurt, and skim milk rather than full-fat milk.

Quick weight loss can actually make fatty liver worse. When you have hepatitis C, crash diets and appetite-suppressing herbs or medications are risky. The solution for fatty liver caused by being overweight is slow, careful dieting supervised by your physician.

Trying to gain weight

A serious effect of hepatitis C or interferon treatment is nausea and lack of appetite, which I discuss in the section "Easing Hep C Symptoms," earlier in this chapter. In some cases, your liver disease may be so severe that you're not getting the nutrition you need. If so, see your doctor and follow her advice about nutritional supplements.

Chapter 12

Avoiding Harmful Substances

● ●

In This Chapter

▶ Understanding why toxins are dangerous

▶ Checking your medications, vitamins, and herbs for safety

▶ Avoiding household and environmental toxins

▶ Saying no to drinking, smoking, and illegal drug use

▶ Seeking help for your addiction

● ●

*W*hy do some people with hepatitis C get end-stage liver disease or liver cancer and others don't? Lots of factors contribute to disease, and things like your age, gender, and how long you've been infected can't be changed. But there's something you can do: Reduce your exposure to potentially dangerous chemicals (toxins).

Some chemicals are known to cause liver damage in certain circumstances. Although this may not be a particular problem for a healthy person, it could be more dangerous for someone with hepatitis C who already has some liver damage.

In this chapter, I describe different types of potential toxins and help you work out a plan to eliminate them, one by one. I also give you some suggestions to deal with addiction and ease your way to a healthier lifestyle. ***A note on terminology:*** When you're talking about your liver, anything you put in your mouth, breathe in, or put on your skin is a chemical to be processed. In this chapter, when I say *chemical* or *drug,* it can refer to substances from food, water, cosmetics, over-the-counter (OTC) or prescribed products, and so on.

Talking about Toxins

You can be exposed to dangerous chemicals from a number of sources. In this chapter, I discuss each of these sources in detail:

- **The environment:** Many chemicals that could be dangerous are in the air, food, or water and are nearly impossible to avoid.

- **Health products:** Health products, including medicines that you may have around the house or use regularly, can be harmful. These include OTC and prescription medications, vitamin and mineral supplements, and herbal products.

- **Household and industrial products:** You likely introduce potentially dangerous chemicals into your home with products such as cleaning agents and bug sprays. At work, you may be exposed to substances, such as solvents, that can be dangerous.

- **Potentially addictive substances:** This category includes alcohol, cigarettes, and street drugs. These addictive substances are dangerous, but they can be very difficult to give up.

The liver is particularly sensitive to chemical damage because it's a clearinghouse for most chemicals that enter the body (for the complete story on the workings of your liver, see Chapter 4). Practically every chemical has the potential to be toxic in the right circumstances.

Anyone, with or without hep C, can get liver damage from drugs or chemicals. But hepatitis C disease, like other liver diseases, can make you more sensitive to liver damage for the following reasons:

- Your liver isn't working so efficiently, so chemicals and drugs that are normally processed by the liver remain in your body longer than expected. When drugs linger in your body, you can get more side effects.

- Your liver already has damage from hepatitis C, so additional damage from a liver toxin can be dangerous and seriously affect liver function.

As you read this chapter, list the potentially toxic substances you use — such as herbal remedies or alcohol — and the toxins in your environment — such as cleaners and pesticides. Make a list in your hep C notebook (see Chapter 5) that includes each dangerous substance from this chapter that you come into contact with. After you make your list, you can work to avoid exposure to some of these chemicals or discuss them with your doctor.

Managing Medications, Supplements, and Herbs

In an awful irony, some of the medications, supplements, and herbs you take to feel better may actually cause harm, especially if you have hep C. Many of these products have the potential for *hepato-toxicity* (liver damage). You may be surprised by what can harm the liver. Then again, you may not be surprised when you consider that the liver metabolizes almost every drug you take. And having liver disease can mean that your body doesn't metabolize medications (and all chemicals) so quickly, which can lead to more side effects.

Adding to the problem is the possibility that different medications you take (including herbs, vitamins, and OTC drugs) and other toxins can interact with one another in a way that's harmful.

The most well-known example is the danger to your liver of taking acetaminophen (Tylenol) at very high doses (more than 2,000 milligrams per day) or taking it with alcohol (see the "Giving Up Alcohol" section, later in this chapter). When taken correctly, acetaminophen is generally safe for use with hep C.

Making safety a priority

Go to your medicine chest and make a list of all OTC medications, prescriptions, vitamins, supplements, and herbs you've taken recently. (If you haven't taken the product recently, you may want to throw it out, especially if it's out of date.) Include the dose for each and run this list by your physician if you haven't cleared everything with her already.

Consider all of your medications, whether they're supplements, herbal remedies, or OTC or prescription drugs. Follow these simple rules to keep yourself safe:

- ✔ Take only substances that are essential and prescribed or recommended by a healthcare practitioner.

- ✔ Make sure your healthcare practitioners are knowledgeable about liver disease (see Chapter 5 for more info on finding and communicating with healthcare providers).

- ✔ Tell all your healthcare providers about every single medication that passes through your lips, nose, or skin and keep them informed of any changes in your medications.

✔ If you develop any reaction to a new or old medication, contact your healthcare provider immediately.

✔ Get all your prescriptions filled at the same pharmacy. This way, the pharmacist has a record of all your medications and can note potential drug interactions and prevent problems.

WARNING!

Don't stop taking any prescribed medication without first checking with your doctor. Some medications must be stopped slowly, and if you go off them on your own, you could risk serious complications.

Watching out for OTC and prescription medications

Over-the-counter drugs have the advantage that you don't need a prescription or health insurance to get them. The disadvantage is that you may not be aware of the potential dangers of certain OTC medications on their own or in combination with other drugs.

You need a doctor's okay for prescription medications, which are also covered by some health insurance policies. An advantage of prescription medications is that you have contact with a pharmacist who can answer questions and look out for drug interactions.

TIP

To check on the possibility of liver problems with any OTC or prescription medications you're taking, your first resource should be your doctor.

Hundreds of medications can potentially cause liver damage or complications. In this section, I list some of the top offenders and those that you're most likely to encounter by generic name (with the brand name in parentheses):

✔ Acarbose (Precose)

✔ Acebutolol (Sectral)

✔ Amiodarone (Cordarone)

✔ Anabolic steroids (Durabolin, Kabolin, and others)

✔ Azathioprine (Imuran)

✔ Birth control pills (progestin and estrogen)

✔ Dantrolene (Dantrium)

✔ Diclofenac (Voltaren and Cataflam)

✔ Estrogen (Premarin)

✔ Felbamate (Felbatol)

✔ Fluconazole and Ketonazole (Diflucan and Nizoral)

✔ Carbamazapine (Tegretol and Atretol)

✔ Gemfibrozil (Lopid)

- ✔ Isoniazid (Laniazid and Nydrazid)
- ✔ Labetalol (Normodyne and Trandate)
- ✔ Leflunomide (Arava)
- ✔ Methotrexate (Maxtrex)
- ✔ Methyldopa (Aldomet)
- ✔ Nefazodone (Serzone)
- ✔ Niacin and nicotinic acid (Niaspan Extended Release Tablets)
- ✔ Nonsteroidal anti-inflammatory drugs
- ✔ Pemoline (Cylert)
- ✔ Phenothiazines (Tindal and Temaril)

- ✔ Phenytoin (Dilantin)
- ✔ Quinidine (Cardoquin and Duraquin)
- ✔ Rifampin (Rifadin)
- ✔ Statins (Zocor and Lipitor)
- ✔ Sulfonamides (antibiotics and derivatives)
- ✔ Tacrine (Cognex)
- ✔ Ticlopidine (Ticlid)
- ✔ Tolcapone (Tasmar)
- ✔ Trovafloxacin (Trovan)
- ✔ Valproic acid (Depakene)
- ✔ Zileutan (Zyflo)

Acetaminophen (or paracetamol in other countries) has been well documented to cause liver damage in high doses or when combined with alcohol. However, it's also frequently the treatment of choice for aches and pains that come with hepatitis C. So take this medication only under the advice of your doctor.

If you like to do your own research, visit `www.medlineplus.gov`, go to the Drug Information section, and find your drug.

Surveying vitamin and mineral supplements

Some folks like to pick supplements on the recommendations of friends or after reading an article. When you have hepatitis C, play it safe and take vitamin and mineral supplements only as recommended by your doctor. Just like the OTC and prescription drugs mentioned earlier, some supplements, especially at high doses, can cause liver problems.

Take any vitamins as prescribed, but don't decide on your own to take even more vitamins. Your doctor will probably prescribe a multivitamin with 100 percent of the RDA (recommended dietary allowance) and maybe other supplements as well. (If you have cirrhosis, you may have vitamin or mineral deficiencies and may need more vitamins or minerals.) Most vitamins and minerals aren't a problem for the liver, but the following three, which are each stored by the liver, can be dangerous if taken at high doses:

- ✔ **Vitamin A:** In high doses, this fat-soluble vitamin that's stored in the liver can be toxic. Don't exceed 5,000 units per day.

- ✔ **Iron:** The liver metabolizes and stores iron. If you have cirrhosis or high levels of iron in your blood, your liver isn't properly metabolizing iron. Excess iron can further damage the liver. Your healthcare provider may advise you to take a multivitamin without iron.

- ✔ **Niacin:** The RDA of niacin (also called nicotinic acid, nicotinamide, and vitamin B3) is 16 milligrams for men, 14 milligrams for women, 17 milligrams for breastfeeding women, and 18 milligrams for pregnant women. High doses of niacin (more than 500 milligrams) can cause liver problems.

Honing in on herbal products

The appeal of using "natural" products that come from the plant kingdom is unquestionable — people throughout the world have been doing so for millennia.

You may want to take herbs for different ailments associated with liver disease and hepatitis C, but just as I warn for medications, vitamins, and minerals, some herbs can damage your liver. Do not self-treat when you have hepatitis C. Don't take any herbal teas, supplements, or *tinctures* (concentrated herbal extracts) — except with the guidance of a liver-knowledgeable herbalist or doctor.

Some herbal tinctures are alcohol based, making them out of the question for recovering alcoholics and others who are staying away from alcohol. Discuss these products with your herbalist and obtain herbs as capsules, teas, or in nonalcohol-based tinctures.

Here's a list of herbs that may damage the liver; avoid them unless advised otherwise by a qualified herbalist:

- ✔ Baikal skullcap or Huang qin *(Scutellaria baicalensis)*

- ✔ Borage *(Borago officinalis)*

- ✔ Chaparral or creosote bush *(Larrea tridentate)*

- ✔ Coltsfoot *(Tussilago farfara)*

- ✔ Comfrey *(Symphytum officinale)*

- ✔ European mistletoe *(Viscum album)*

✔ Germander *(Teucrium chamaedrys)*

✔ Golden ragwort *(Senecio aureus)*

✔ Groundsel *(Senecio longilobusvulgaris)*

✔ Heliotropium *(Heliotropium europaeum)*

✔ Hemp agrimony *(Eupatorium cannibinum)*

✔ Jin Bu Huan *(Lycopocium serratum)*

✔ Kava *(Piper methysticum)*

✔ Margosa or neem oil *(Azadirachta indica)*

✔ Pennyroyal oil *(Mentha pulegium)*

✔ Sassafras *(Sassafras ablidum)*

✔ Senna *(Senna alexandrina)*

✔ Skullcap *(Scuttellaria lateriflora)*

✔ Tansy ragwort *(Senecio jacoboea)*

✔ Uva ursi *(Arctostaphylos uva-ursi)*

✔ Valerian *(Valeriana officinalis)*

Cleaning Up Household, Industrial, and Environmental Toxins

Household, industrial, and environmental toxins are usually referred to as toxic chemicals. *Toxicity* is a measure of the danger of the chemical to the liver, kidney, heart, or brain.

Listing types of chemical toxins

Some chemicals are toxic to the liver, either by causing chemical hepatitis or by affecting liver enzyme levels (which I discuss in Chapter 7). Toxic or dangerous chemicals can also be carcinogenic (cause cancer), affect your immune system, or hurt other organs, like your brain or kidneys.

Chemicals that are toxic to your liver are in your home, garden, workplace, and just about anywhere in the environment. You can be exposed by inhaling toxic fumes, getting some on your skin, or accidentally getting some in your mouth or eyes. Here's a list of some common types of toxic chemicals you may be exposed to:

✔ **Pesticides and insecticides:** Chemicals that are meant to kill critters have a good chance of also being toxic for humans. These are found in homes as bug sprays for indoor and outdoor use. There might also be residues on your food.

✔ **Herbicides:** These chemicals are used to control weeds and can also be toxic.

✔ **Household cleaning products:** Agents such as air fresheners, carpet cleaners, drain cleaners, and furniture polish can contain dangerous chemicals.

✔ **Solvents:** Solvents are extremely dangerous because you can breathe them in or get exposure through your skin. Solvents are found in the home in products such as carpet glues, cleaning fluids, paint, paint thinners, primers, and wood sealers. Industrial solvents include adhesives, epoxy resins, hardeners, lacquers, and mastics (asphalt or coal-tar).

Because you probably have at least some of these chemicals around your house, you need to know how to use them safely, which I describe in the next section.

Putting safety first

Think about it: If a chemical is capable of killing bugs or plants or erasing oily deposits, what do you think that chemical could do to your body? I would add that if it smells horrible and you feel sick from being around it, well, that's a sign of a chemical you shouldn't be around, isn't it?

Assume that all cleaners, pesticides, and solvents are unsafe so that you use them with caution, if at all. Follow these guidelines when using chemicals around the house:

✔ Limit the amount you use and how often you use the chemicals.

✔ Read labels carefully.

✔ Follow directions exactly.

✔ Don't mix chemicals.

✔ Avoid breathing the chemicals by keeping the area well ventilated and wearing a protective respiratory mask.

✔ Cover your skin with clothing and wear rubber or latex gloves so that the chemicals don't touch your skin.

✔ Wash your hands and clothing after using chemicals.

If you or a family member ingests a chemical toxin or gets some on the skin or in the eyes, call your doctor or 911 immediately.

Keeping your home toxin free

Make your home a safe place where you can rest assured that no noxious chemical agents are lurking. Try some of these suggestions for a home clean home:

✔ Take an inventory of the cleansers, insecticides, pesticides, and other chemicals in your house, garage, and shed. Read the labels and very carefully dispose of old or dangerous products.

✔ Shop with your liver in mind. Read product labels carefully and avoid introducing new toxins into your home as possible.

✔ Clean without fumigating yourself:

• Buy nontoxic cleaning products (found in health food stores).

• Make your own cleaning products (try vinegar and baking soda) and use old-fashioned muscle power combined with scrubbing brushes or steel wool.

✔ Keep away pests without hurting yourself:

• Try organic gardening and lawn care (check out *Organic Gardening For Dummies,* by Ann Whitman and the editors at the National Gardening Association, published by Wiley).

• Clean your kitchen and garden of all crumbs or debris that can attract critters.

• Try nonchemical methods of bug control, such as electronic deterrents or biological control.

• If you must use chemical warfare against pests, wear protective clothing and gloves.

✔ Beware of sprays of any kind — most have dangerous chemicals that you could accidentally inhale.

✔ Try to keep cigarette smoke out of your home. Secondhand smoke is a carcinogen. If there's still smoking going on in your house or pollution from outside, invest in air purifiers that use a filtration system.

I also discuss using pesticide-free food (organic) and purified water in Chapter 11.

In your bathroom, you may have lotions, potions, and cosmetics with possibly toxic or irritating chemicals. If you have sensitive skin, you're allergic to certain products, or you're generally concerned about your skin-care or shampooing products, speak to your doctor, pharmacist, or herbalist. And check out the cosmetic information page on the Food and Drug Administration Web site by going to www.cfsan.fda.gov and clicking on the Cosmetics link.

Taking care of business: Toxic workplaces

Some workplaces can be toxic (I'm talking about chemicals, not your colleagues or supervisors). If you work at a gas station, dry cleaner, chemical plant, art studio, or other location where you face constant exposure to solvents or other poisonous chemicals, talk to your doctor about your situation and what steps you should take to deal with the problem.

For more information about toxins in the workplace, contact the U.S. Occupational Safety and Health Administration (OSHA) — the Web site is www.osha.gov — or the National Institute for Occupational Safety and Health (NIOSH) — www.cdc.gov/niosh.

Your options include changing your job tasks or even leaving your job if you can't avoid daily exposure to danger.

Quitting Smoking

Cigarette smoke contains more than 4,000 chemicals, and more than 50 of them are known to cause cancer (carcinogen). As your risk of liver cancer increases with hepatitis C infection, smoking is even more dangerous.

But cigarettes aren't the only culprits in this category. All types of smoking — cigars, pipes, or even marijuana — carry a danger to your liver because of the additives and dangerous chemicals that are produced in the smoke and transported through the lungs to the bloodstream to the liver. There's no escape! Most chemicals, no matter what their entry point, end up in the liver.

Protect your liver and quit smoking today. See your healthcare professional for help. You can also check in with the folks at the American Lung Association (www.lungusa.org) for more information on kicking the habit and take part in their free online smoking-cessation program. And for more info on the dangers of cigarettes, check out www.ash.org.

Giving Up Alcohol

Whether you're a regular drinker or social sipper, giving up alcohol belongs near the top of your to-do list if you have hepatitis C. Some folks will say that a single glass of alcohol can reduce stress or the risk of heart disease. But when you have hepatitis C, those potential benefits don't matter. Consuming any kind of alcohol provides a risk to your liver that's greater than any possible benefit.

If you still need convincing, consider the following list of reasons to eliminate alcohol from your diet:

✔ Alcohol consumption can lead to fatty liver condition, acute and chronic hepatitis, cirrhosis, and end-stage liver failure.

✔ Studies on alcohol use and hep C progression have found a relationship between heavy drinking and the development of fibrosis. Studies aren't clear about how lower levels of drinking might affect hep C.

✔ In lab studies, alcohol stimulates the growth of the hep C virus.

✔ Alcohol taken with other drugs, such as acetaminophen (see the "Watching out for OTC and prescription medications" section, earlier in the chapter), makes the effect on the liver much worse.

✔ Alcoholics may not be able to participate in interferon therapy (check out Chapter 8). Laboratory studies show that alcohol reduces the effects of interferon.

✔ Heavy alcohol consumption will keep you off the waiting list for a liver transplant (see Chapter 9).

So what were your reasons for drinking?

Defining drinking types and identifying a problem

Eliminating alcohol from your life may be easier if you know your drinking style. Your doctor will inevitably ask you lots of questions about your drinking. Be truthful. This information enables you and your healthcare practitioner to devise the most effective treatment plan possible. (I cover how to work with your doctor in Chapter 5.)

When adding up how much you drink, count one drink as the following:

- 12 ounces of beer
- 5 ounces of wine
- 1½ ounces of liquor

Use this rough guide to the drinking types to figure out where you fit in. Amounts can vary, depending on your weight and gender.

- **Abstainer (nondrinker):** Doesn't drink at all.

- **Social drinker:** Likes to drink but could easily give it up and may be a light, moderate, or heavy social drinker.

  - **Light social drinker:** One drink or less per week.

  - **Moderate social drinker:** One to two drinks per night.

  - **Heavy social drinker:** More than one or two drinks per night.

- **Problem drinker or alcoholic:** Has lost the ability to control his drinking. It doesn't matter whether drinking is moderate or heavy or occurs only during *binges* (heavy drinking at intervals). If you suspect that you fall within this category, please seek help as described in the section "Getting Help for Alcohol or Drug Addiction," later in this chapter.

Alcohol can damage the body, whether you drink socially or alcoholically. If you have hepatitis C, avoid it. The difference is that a social drinker can usually stop, whereas an alcoholic needs help. If you believe you're a social drinker, check out the "Socializing without drinking" section, later in the chapter.

There's no shame in having a drinking problem. Alcoholism is a disease shared by millions of Americans, and many have obtained help. Here's a list of questions to see whether you may be a problem drinker or alcoholic:

- Are you worried about your drinking?

- Do you drink alone?

- Do you drink to numb your feelings?

- Does your drinking affect your work?

- Does your drinking worry your family or friends?

- Have you tried to control your drinking?

- Do you ever forget what happened while you were drinking?

- Do you get sick with headaches or hangovers after drinking?

If you answered yes to one or more of these questions, you may have a problem with alcohol. Seek professional help and see the section on "Getting Help for Alcohol or Drug Addiction," later in the chapter.

Socializing without drinking

People in movies, on television, at parties, on the beach, by the pool, at the club, and at the bar all seem to be drinking up a storm. You may wonder how the heck you can give up such wonderful stuff. But a closer look at the Hollywood version of drinking yields tales of alcoholism and woe. And for people with hep C, the potential danger to your liver outweighs any possible benefit.

For social drinkers, here are some tips to get through life without drinking. If you're a problem drinker, seek professional help.

- ✔ Keep your house alcohol free, if possible.

- ✔ Enlist help from your support network (see Chapter 14).

- ✔ Use relaxation techniques such as meditation and yoga (see Chapter 13).

If people ask why you're not drinking, you don't have to tell them about your hepatitis unless you want to. Nowadays, many people give up alcohol for health or diet reasons. You're among a growing number of people who choose not to drink. Try one of the smooth nonalcoholic drinks listed in Chapter 11. Holding a wineglass filled with club soda and a twist of lemon will help you feel like part of the merriment and not obviously different.

Dealing with Dangerous Street Drugs

Sharing equipment when injecting or snorting drugs is one of the ways to acquire hepatitis C. If you've given up illegal drugs, hats off to you. If you're still hooked, check out the "Getting Help for Alcohol or Drug Addiction" section, later in the chapter. Even if you already have hepatitis C, you're endangering yourself by continuing to use drugs.

Illegal drugs can accelerate the hepatitis C disease because they cause the following problems:

✔ Reduce your immune response.

✔ Expose you to toxins from the impurities added to street drugs.

✔ Impair your ability to respond to treatment (if you can even get treatment while using drugs).

✔ Eliminate your ability to receive a liver transplant until you are off illicit drugs for six months.

✔ Increase your risk of getting superinfected with hepatitis B, HIV, or another type of hepatitis C by sharing paraphernalia associated with injection or snorting drug use. See Chapter 2 for information on transmission and protecting others from hep C.

With street drugs, the drug itself or the method of intake, whether it's injecting, snorting, or smoking, can be dangerous. Cocaine has been shown to directly cause liver toxicity. Whether you smoke, snort, or inject cocaine, you're hurting your liver. Snorting cocaine through a shared straw can spread hepatitis C because doing so causes frequent nosebleeds.

The bottom line is to stop using or at least reduce your use of all illicit or street drugs. I know — if it were so easy, you'd have stopped using long ago. Do it differently this time and get help. And give yourself lots of TLC (tender loving care) as you learn to live drug free.

Getting Help for Alcohol or Drug Addiction

If you can't stop drinking or using drugs on your own, don't lose hope! Here's a plan of action:

✔ See your doctor or healthcare practitioner. He can refer you to alcohol or drug treatment and suggest a detoxification plan to help you through alcohol and/or drug withdrawal.

✔ Call the National Drug and Alcohol Treatment Referral Routing Service (Center for Substance Abuse Treatment) at 800-662-HELP (800-662-4357) to find treatment programs in your community.

✔ Contact Alcoholics Anonymous (AA) or Narcotics Anonymous (NA) for info on their 12-step programs and to find out how to attend a meeting near your home. Check your local phone book for contact info or check out either organization online by logging on to www.alcoholics-anonymous.org or www.na.org. Both sites provide contact information for groups and meetings in your area. Here is some general info on these programs:

- The 12-step approach helps you recover from addiction by changing your attitudes and behavior.

- You'll meet and get support from others who have successfully given up their substance of choice — one day at a time.

- AA and NA are not religious programs, but they do use a spiritual approach. You can be an atheist or agnostic and still get help.

Recognizing that the drink or drug you first took to feel good is now killing you is shocking and scary. Don't numb that feeling. You deserve to live and have a good life.

Chapter 13

Moving and Grooving to Reduce Stress and Feel Better

Stress happens — to everyone. But when you're facing a chronic illness like hepatitis C, the stress can be more pronounced, and its effects can be more harmful. Hepatitis C also comes with its own set of physical complications and problems. But whether you're experiencing the mental, emotional, or physical effects of stress, or you're fighting fatigue and anxiety, adding some exercise or movement to your routine can help you feel better. In this chapter, I define stress and its role in your life but quickly move on to simple tips to reduce that stress. Then I describe multiple techniques to soothe your body, mind, and spirit.

Explore the options in this chapter and pick a few that work for you. You can try exercises like walking or swimming or the more subtle but powerful ancient movements of T'ai Chi, Qigong, or Yoga. Or consider visiting a qualified bodywork practitioner who can help you relieve muscle tension and relax. You can even try not moving! Practice calmness by using breathing, relaxation, meditation, or visualizing techniques. I cover all of these ideas — and more.

Getting a Handle on Stress and Hepatitis C

We live in a world where lots of people are stressed out. So what exactly is this stress that everyone talks about? One way of defining stress is the *body's response to a change or challenge.* The change or challenge that causes the stress is called a *stressor,* which could be anything from the freezing temperature outside, to a new medicine you're taking, to an attack dog that's charging after you! Stress is so important that I define different types — short or long term and physical or emotional stress — in the following sections.

Acute versus chronic stress

During the stress response, energy is diverted from your immune, digestive, and reproductive systems and focused on giving you a supreme burst of energy.

The body is designed to deal with short-term (acute) stress. When a stressor first arrives — in the form of an attack dog, for example — your body takes most of its energy reserves to fight or help you run like the devil to save your life. When the dog is gone, your body returns to normal because you no longer need the extra energy diverted to save your life.

In modern times, we have a lot of long-term (chronic) stress. These are challenges that don't go away and keep us stressed out for long periods of time. These stressors can range from a difficult boss or financial worries to a long-term chronic illness, like hepatitis C. This fight-or-flight biological response was better suited to the precarious lives of cave dwellers and their many physical threats.

The problem with long-term stress is that your body doesn't get to go back to a nonstressed state. In modern times, when mundane things like traffic jams and deadlines trigger stress, it's not so useful to lose precious energy in response to these almost-constant stressors. When you have hepatitis C, the last thing you want is for energy to be taken away from your immune system.

Physical stress

A healthy body is in an exquisite state of balance called *homeostasis.* Any disruption to your body from an injury or an illness causes physical stress. The hepatitis C virus causes physical stress just by being a foreigner in your body and making your immune system go into attack mode.

Likewise, to keep its balance, your body needs proper amounts and types of nutrition, rest, movement, fresh air, and warmth. Too much of anything (including food, exercise, and heat) and the wrong types of things (such as polluted air, junk food, and dangerous drugs) also cause stress.

If a physical stress is short term — like missing some sleep on exam night or having an occasional ice cream — the body can usually recover. But with long-term physical stress, like not sleeping for weeks or smoking cigarettes for years, the body has a more difficult time regaining its balance.

Emotional and mental stress

Much of our modern stress comes from mental and emotional anxiety. Pressures and worries to get to work on time, make deadlines, pay bills, get your kids into college, and so on can trigger an emotional stress response. With hep C, you probably have worries related to one or more of the following things:

- Overall health
- Sexual interest or ability (due to hepatitis C or medication)
- Financial situation
- Work hours, job conditions, or the job itself
- Lifestyle (diet, alcohol consumption, smoking)

And I'm sure you can add a few more worries of your own. Emotional stress is a funny thing because any type of change, even good change, can be stressful. Think of the stress that can accompany the first year of marriage or bringing home a new baby!

Linking stress and illness

Illness is a major challenge to the normal workings of your body and causes stress in different ways. The physical aspects of the stress caused by hep C are pretty straightforward and include the interaction among the following:

- **The hepatitis C virus:** The virus is growing and making proteins inside your body, which affects your immune system, your liver cells, and other parts of your body.

✔ **The immune system:** Your immune system is now in attack mode because it senses danger from the hep C virus.

✔ **Your liver:** The liver has trouble doing its job when the war between the hep C virus and the immune system is being fought in its midst.

These physical components of hepatitis C virus infection interact with the emotional aspects of stress. Anxiety, fatigue, and depression are common emotional components of hepatitis C. (I delve into depression in hepatitis C in Chapter 14 and discuss anxiety and fatigue in the following sections.)

Because stress hormones affect the brain and the body, stress affects your mind and your body. Whether you have physical or emotional stress, remember that stress of one type can add to the stress of another type, so stress itself is stressful! It's a two-way street: Physical stress can lead to emotional stress, and emotional stress can lead to physical stress. And both play a role in lessening your body's ability to protect itself against hep C.

If you try the self-help tips described in this chapter and still suffer from anxiety, fatigue, or depression, discuss these problems with your doctor. In some cases, your doctor may be able to make further suggestions or prescribe or change your medication.

Looking at anxiety and tension

Anxiety is a type of emotional stress based on worrying thoughts. You know it's anxiety when your thoughts start with the words *what if.* Anxiety is part of a natural fear response to a threat or challenge to your life. But when anxiety reaches a peak, that's called a *panic attack,* in which your biological stress response really goes haywire.

Muscle tension is one symptom of anxiety, and you may have sore shoulders, neck, or back. The pain of being tense can lead to headaches and difficulty sleeping.

Fitting fatigue into the picture

Fatigue is probably the most commonly reported symptom of hep C. I'm not talking about just drowsiness, which is a feeling of sleepiness or needing more sleep. *Fatigue* is the term for feelings of low energy, weariness, or being tired.

Researchers haven't been able to prove whether the fatigue from hepatitis C is due directly to the virus or results from the emotional response to and stress of being ill. This is a chicken-and-egg question: Which came first? If you're suffering from fatigue, however, all that really matters is that you want to feel better soon.

Reducing stress —
one way or another

Because stress is so pervasive in modern life and potentially harmful — even more so for folks with a chronic illness like hep C — I have lots of suggestions for ways to deal with stress and diminish its effects on your health and your life in general. Pick the ones that feel most useful to you.

The key to keeping stress from hurting you is in your *reaction* to it. Practice some of these techniques, and you'll be humming or giggling instead of stressing out.

Taking care of body basics

You can start fighting stress by taking care of your body:

- ✓ **Exercise.** Find out about the different types of exercise you may want to consider in the section "Considering types of exercise," later in the chapter.

- ✓ **Regularly eat nutritious meals.** I discuss this topic in Chapter 11.

- ✓ **Get enough quality sleep.** When you have hep C, you may have trouble sleeping. For tips on sleep, see Chapter 21.

Keeping the physical body in good shape gives you more resilience to deal with stress. Remember to avoid physical stressors like breathing polluted air, smoking cigarettes, taking street drugs, and drinking alcohol (see Chapter 12).

Respecting your limits and needs

An important part of emotional stress is the feeling of not having control over your life. You may feel that having hepatitis C has put you on a roller coaster that you don't know how to stop. Here are some ways to bring back some of your personal power:

- ✓ **Say no.** One of the easiest ways to get stressed is to take on too many tasks. Recognize your limits and accept them.

- ✓ **Ask for help.** Don't be afraid to ask for help. Ask your family and friends, social service workers, doctors, fellow support group members, and neighbors for help when you need it (see Chapter 14 for more on support).

- ✓ **Get information.** The more you know about your options with hep C, the more empowered and less stressed you'll feel. That's what this book is all about, and Chapter 22 contains other sources of information.

✔ **Keep your health info organized.** A hep C notebook may seem like a stressful task initially, but in the long run, organization will make your life easier (see Chapter 5 for info on setting up such a notebook). Also keep your health insurance claims and medical bills organized in one place (see Chapter 16).

Relaxing your body and easing your thoughts

Stress and anxiety make your body tense, tense, tense. Your worries may be keeping you from a restful sleep, but engaging in body-based therapies can help you relax. In the "Experiencing Body-Based Therapies" section, later in the chapter, I cover many of these forms of relief.

Enjoying life

If you're not feeling well, you may forget to do the things you love. I'm reminding you now to remember the pleasures of life, which can distract you from your pain and may even make you feel better.

✔ **Listen to music.** Music therapy can bring you some joy. Find a CD or radio station that plays music that soothes you, whether it's jazz, classical, or folk. Other types of sounds, such as waves, sometimes also have a calming effect.

✔ **Engage your creative side.** Everyone has creativity waiting to be expressed. Lose yourself in drawing, taking photographs, or sewing a piece of patchwork. Or maybe you enjoy dancing, playing the piano, cooking a meal, or arranging a few flowers in a vase.

✔ **Connect with nature.** Try to experience nature. Whether it's the beach, a forest, or the mountains, get outdoors and breathe some fresh air. Or simply go to your backyard or a local park and notice the different types of trees and flowers

✔ **Focus on spirituality.** Whether you belong to an organized religion or you have your own way of expressing the divine, find a way to bring the sacred to your everyday life: Light a candle, say the prayers of your particular faith, or make up your own prayers. I offer suggestions for meditation, which can be used as one way to get in touch with your spiritual side, in "Quieting the mind with meditation," later in this chapter.

✔ **Play with your pets.** Research has shown that spending time with your furry friends helps reduce stress. They're less stressed than humans are, so they can help you relax, especially when they start purring or wagging their tails.

✔ **Spend time with family and friends.** Have you stayed in contact with close family and friends? In today's world, it's easy to isolate yourself or get too busy to keep in touch with others.

But calling an old friend or inviting a family member to dinner can give you a real pick-me-up. Your family and friends may want to read Chapter 19, which I wrote just for them.

✔ **Enjoy intimacy.** Everyone needs to feel connected and close to loved ones, but that can be hard for people with hepatitis C. I cover communicating with your loved one and sexual issues in Chapter 15.

✔ **Find humor:** Laughter is a known healer. Find a funny movie or interact with pets or children who have a sense of humor.

Exercising Your Fitness Options

Moving around can be the solution to the fatigue, stress, and achy joints that often come with hep C. Your body is meant to be moving in some way or another.

Why exercise?

When you're tired, exercise is probably the last thing on your mind. Think again. Exercise actually has the ability to make you feel less tired — no, I'm not kidding. Exercise offers the following benefits:

✔ Boosts your energy levels

✔ Improves the functioning of your immune system

✔ Helps control your weight

✔ Helps you sleep better

✔ Improves your endurance

✔ Increases strength in your muscles

✔ Relieves stress and anxiety

✔ Enhances your mood

All those rewards for a relatively small investment of your time! The trick is to put on your sneakers, drive to the gym, or schedule some time to watch that exercise video. Whatever amount or type of exercise you can muster will help you feel better.

Sticking with an exercise program

Like many a New Year's resolution, starting a new exercise regimen is easier than keeping it going. In this section, I focus on tips to help you achieve continued success with your program.

Before starting any exercise program, check with your doctor. After getting the green light, if you experience any symptoms during exercise — such as chest pain, breathlessness, nausea, lightheadedness, or extreme fatigue — pay another visit to your healthcare provider.

If you have cirrhosis or portal hypertension (see Chapter 4), you may need to avoid certain exercises or positions. Talk with your doctor for specific advice.

Here are some suggestions to increase the likelihood that you'll stick to your fitness routine:

- ✔ **Determine your goals.** Depending on your level of fitness, your hep C symptoms, and the condition of your liver and heart, you may have any or all of the following goals when you start an exercise:

  - Increase the mobility of your joints

  - Ease your aches and pains

  - Sleep better

  - Have more energy

  - Lose a couple inches around your waist

  - Become more fit

- ✔ **Get professional advice.** Your healthcare professional, a personal trainer, or qualified instructors in the exercise of your choice are good sources to contact. If you're new to exercise in general, you're beginning a new exercise regimen, or you're coming back to exercise after an illness, a pro can help guide you and devise a plan that fits your health and exercise goals.

- ✔ **Start gently and build slowly.** Don't overdo it, especially at first. Start with 5 minutes and work up to 20 to 30 minutes of exercise per day for 3 days a week. You can then increase the number of days or amount of time if that's appropriate for you. Too much exercise can tire you out and lead to exhaustion. Too little exercise, and you won't get as much benefit.

- ✔ **Choose a time that's convenient.** If you work out at a time that's good for *you,* you're more likely to exercise. Many people exercise in the morning to avoid procrastination later in the day. On the other hand, your body may be suppler later in the day.

- ✔ **Pick an exercise you enjoy.** If you dislike an activity, you aren't likely to keep it up for long. Consider activities such as working in the garden, dancing, walking your dog, or playing with children as ways to work exercise into your day.

Considering types of exercise

Exercise is divided into three categories: aerobic, strength training, and stretching. Most exercises or types of movement fall into more than one of these categories. Your exercise program should optimally provide a balance of all three.

Aerobic activities

Aerobic means "with air" or "using oxygen," and if done with a certain intensity, these exercises will make you huff and puff. Aerobic exercise helps you burn fat and decrease the risks of heart disease and cancer. The following are the more common aerobic exercises:

- ✔ **Walking:** By far, walking is the easiest, most popular, and least costly sport to pursue. All you need are good-quality walking shoes, a jacket for rain or cold, sunglasses, and sunscreen. Start by walking around your block and work your way up to longer walks. To start a walking program, check out *Fitness Walking For Dummies,* by Liz Neporent (published by Wiley).

- ✔ **Swimming:** Get your bathing suit and goggles and head for the nearest pool. Check out the local public pool; the YMCA; or private pools at a swim club, country club, or neighborhood clubhouse. If you decide that swimming is your thing, you can often obtain a season pass or yearly membership.

- ✔ **Bicycling:** Bicycling can be fun, and you may even be able to cycle to work, the library, or the supermarket. When you go out on the road, put on a helmet, watch out for vehicles, and obey safety rules. If you use a stationary bicycle at home or at the gym, you can watch television or read a book at the same time.

- ✔ **Low-impact aerobics classes or videos:** Visit your local YMCA or fitness club or rent or buy videotapes or DVDs of experienced fitness instructors. You can also borrow them for free from your public library.

Strength training

Keeping your muscles toned and strong is the purpose of strengthening exercises. Benefits include boosting your metabolism, decreasing the risks of osteoporosis, building joint strength, providing balance, and aiding posture. You can use light weights or strength-training machines at home or head to the gym to work out under supervision.

Stretching

Performing stretching exercises will increase your flexibility and can give you some relief from aches and pains. Yoga is a great way to develop flexibility, and T'ai Chi also works on improving flexibility (I cover these options in the section "Using Mind-Body Techniques," later in the chapter). Or try Pilates or other stretching classes or tapes to stay supple.

Using Mind-Body Techniques

All exercise of your physical body also affects your mind — because the body and mind are intricately connected. But some systems of movement are designed as a whole system of wellness for the body and mind, and even for the spirit. The centuries-old exercises described here have been designed to align the body and mind toward health.

Yearning for Yoga

Yoga has been practiced in India for thousands of years and now is enjoyed by millions of people around the world. Yoga is what you make of it and can be used as simply another type of fitness exercise or as a healthy approach to life. Yoga isn't a religion, and people of any background can study Yoga.

The beauty of Yoga is that you can benefit from any of the aspects of it: breathing, physical postures, meditation, or relaxation. Most people who study Yoga today focus on the *postures,* or positions, that are meant to maximize flexibility and stimulate the mind, body, and spirit. Postures can be performed sitting, standing, or lying down. Many Yoga classes end with a period of relaxation and/or meditation.

If you're a beginning yogi (male) or yogini (female), take a class with a qualified teacher to learn how to move properly. You can also purchase Yoga videos. Get recommendations for videos or classes from friends or folks in your hep C support group.

Don't compare yourself with the other people in your Yoga class. Yoga is an individual pursuit, and keep in mind that you're working with *your* body. Even though Yoga can be gentle, you can injure yourself if you push too hard or use the wrong postures.

Energizing with T'ai Chi

T'ai Chi (pronounced *tie-chee*) is a gentle martial art that has been practiced in China for thousands of years. T'ai Chi is a set of graceful movements that flow into one another that you perform while standing. T'ai Chi is a low-impact activity and can be performed without stressing your joints.

This ancient Chinese martial art is considered a perfect balance between yin and yang — opposite forces (see Chapter 10 for discussion of yin and yang). In T'ai Chi, you slow down so that your awareness increases, and each movement you make is deliberate and powerful. T'ai chi uses exercises that

- ✔ Combine body and mind
- ✔ Use mindful breathing
- ✔ Focus on vital energy called *chi*

Chi is energy that's sometimes spelled *qi* (as in the Chinese practice Qigong); both spellings are pronounced *chee,* as in *cheese.* Chi within the body flows through meridians or channels (also described with acupuncture in Chapter 10). Chi also exists in the universe around us, in living plants and animals as well as inanimate objects.

You can learn T'ai Chi by attending a class or watching a video, and then you can practice in a group or on your own. In China, millions of people practice T'ai Chi daily, and T'ai Chi classes are held in parks around the world. See the sidebar "T'ai Chi and immunity" in this chapter for more information on the subject.

Technically, T'ai Chi is one of the many forms of Qigong. T'ai Chi and Qigong can be practiced separately or in combination. Qigong is a series of shorter exercises that involve movement, breathing, and relaxation. Qigong is a profound way to move energy in your body and is used for healing. A master of Qigong can use this energy to heal others.

T'ai Chi and immunity

An exciting research finding (reported in the September/October 2003 issue of the journal *Psychosomatic Medicine*) found that T'ai Chi could boost immunity to a virus infection. Researchers studied a type of T'ai Chi, called T'ai Chi Chih, for 15 weeks in older people in California. When they were tested afterward, the people who had performed the T'ai Chi had improved scores on a test of immunity against the virus that causes chicken pox and shingles.

The researchers who performed the study (Michael R. Irwin, Jennifer L. Pike, Jason C. Cole, and Michael N. Oxman) believe that T'ai Chi probably increases immunity for other viruses, not just for the virus in their study. Further studies will look at how long the increased immunity lasts. If T'ai Chi can increase immunity to one type of virus, it could possibly help with immunity to the hepatitis C virus, too. More studies are needed to prove this connection between T'ai Chi and other types of immunity.

Experiencing Body-Based Therapies

If your muscles are achy or tense, which can happen when you have hepatitis C, or you just feel the need for some healing touch, find a qualified, experienced practitioner for body work. It's a treat for the body, mind, and spirit.

To find a massage therapist or reiki practitioner, ask your health-care practitioners, friends, or family for recommendations. Some health insurance plans now cover alternative treatments such as massage. Check with your insurance provider and get a referral from your primary care physician, if necessary. If you don't have access to insurance coverage for these therapies, some practitioners use sliding scales for payment.

Massage therapy

Having a massage may seem like a luxury, but it can really help you feel better quicker. A trained and licensed massage therapist uses her hands to knead your muscles. Primarily used for relaxation, a massage can reduce tension, increase circulation, and help ease achy joints. Types of massage include the following:

- ✓ **Swedish massage:** This manipulation of muscles and joints is the most common type of massage and was originally developed in Sweden.

- ✓ **Deep-tissue massage:** The practitioner really goes deep into your muscles to ease out knots of tension.

- ✓ **Hot-stone massage:** This massage uses heated smooth stones to send warmth to tight muscles and as aids to work through your muscles. The warm stones help you feel nurtured during the massage.

- ✓ **Aromatherapy:** The practitioner mixes healing essential oils, such as lavender or rosemary, with the body oil or lotion that's rubbed into your body. This is smelly in a good way.

The above types of massages require you to be undressed, with your body draped with a sheet, while the practitioner uses oils or lotions to massage or stroke your body. The practices below are performed when you are fully clothed (except for shoes) and don't use oil:

- ✓ **Shiatsu:** The practitioner presses on your pressure points to help in relaxation and healing; Shiatsu originated in Japan.

✔ **Reflexology:** The practitioner presses on specific points on your feet (or hands) that correspond to different parts of your body.

Different practitioners may use one or more of these techniques in the same session. Tell your practitioner about any aches and pains, relax on the massage table, and enjoy!

If your family wants to know what to get you for your birthday or the holidays, suggest a session or two of body work. Also, you may get a discount if you book a few sessions at once.

Energy work

Whereas a massage therapist manipulates your physical body to help you relax, an energy worker helps you relax on an energetic level. Not everyone grooves with this technique, but it works — trust me! Energy work is preferable to massage if you don't want to be massaged or get undressed. It's possible to do some types of energy work with hands near but not touching the body.

The beliefs behind energy work are that the body is made of energy and that illness or disease is the result of an energy imbalance. Whether you believe in that or not, energy work can result in profound relaxation, which lets the body heal itself. Two examples of energy work are:

✔ **Reiki** (pronounced ray-key) is a form of hands-on energy healing that originated in Japan. The practitioner is channeling universal energy to you through her hands. Check out www.reiki.org to find out more about reiki.

✔ **Therapeutic touch** was originally developed by a nurse and a healer and has specific treatments for different ailments. The practitioner uses his hands to help unblock your energy. *Healing touch* is another form of treatment that developed from therapeutic touch. Check out www.healingtouch.net to find out more about this type of healing work.

Practitioners (some of whom are registered nurses and medical doctors) carry out therapeutic touch and reiki in some hospital and hospice settings. A practitioner may use energy work in conjunction with a complementary practice, such as massage.

Chinese medicine also has forms of energy work: Qigong and acupuncture/acupressure, which work with the energy meridians. See the "Energizing with T'ai Chi" section, earlier in this chapter, and Chapter 10 for more information.

Calming Yourself

You may not be able to get to a practitioner to help you relax. So here are some techniques you can use in your home or even at work on a daily basis. When your body and mind are relaxed, your body stands a better chance of healing itself.

Relaxing the body

Anxiety and tension can lead to muscle aches, headaches, and trouble sleeping. You can use the technique of progressive relaxation in bed or at the end of an exercise session to help you relax. *Progressive relaxation* is a method of releasing tension in your body by focusing on one body part at a time — that's where the "progressive" part comes in. You might find a tape or practice relaxation in a Yoga class. Here's a brief example of a progressive relaxation technique. Take each step slowly:

1. **Lie down on your back and make yourself comfortable.**

2. **Take a few deep breaths.**

3. **Starting with your feet, relax your left foot, followed by your right foot, your left leg, and then your right leg.**

4. **Move your concentration up to your buttocks and pelvis and then on to your abdomen and lower back, chest, and shoulders.**

5. **Finally, concentrate on relaxing your left hand and arm, right hand and arm, and then your neck and head.**

Another version of this exercise calls for tightening each part of the body as you think of it and then relaxing that part. Enjoy the feeling of peace and ease. Breathe. The more you practice relaxation, the easier it becomes.

Focusing on your breath

The breath is essential for life. It forms a cycle of *in* with life-giving oxygen and *out* with poisonous carbon dioxide. Many forms of exercise (such as Pilates) and mind-body techniques (including T'ai Chi and Yoga) have specific instructions for breathing.

When you're stressed or nervous, you may find that your breathing changes. The breath is a constant and gentle reminder of the flow of life. Focusing on breathing is a way to slow down and relax. Breathing techniques can be used anywhere, anytime: at home, in the doctor's office, in the car, on the telephone, or at work. When you focus on your breathing or perform a breathing exercise, you're consciously relaxing your breath, which aids in overall relaxation and allows your body to get the oxygen it needs.

Here are some ideas for breathing exercises. Sit up straight in a chair, close your eyes, and focus on your breathing:

- ✔ **Pay attention to your breath.** That's it. Just paying attention to each breath is a way of relaxation.

- ✔ **Take deeper breaths.** When you fully release the stale air from your lungs, you create more room for oxygenated air to enter.

- ✔ **Hold the air briefly in between in and out breaths.** Try breathing in through your nose, holding your breath, and then whooshing the air out through your mouth two or three times.

Make sure you're breathing fresh air when doing breathing exercises. Buddhist and Yoga practices of meditation both focus on the breath. If you go to Yoga classes, you'll find out about breathing there, too.

Quieting the mind with meditation

One dictionary defines meditation as thinking about something, but the practice of *meditation* is actually to not think or, if you do think, to focus on something peaceful or spiritual.

Mediation is used to quiet the mind, achieve inner peace, and connect with the universal spirit. Practicing meditation to quiet the mind reduces some of the thoughts and worries that lead to stress and anxiety. You can gain peace and bring in your spirit for renewed energy to help you heal from hep C. Many religions have specific meditation practices. Here are some common ways to achieve the state of meditation:

- ✔ **Go to a quiet place.** Turn off your telephone, close your door, and shut down the computer.

- ✔ **Set aside a period of time.** It can be a few minutes or an hour.

- ✔ **Be comfortable.** In some Buddhist and Yoga practices, you sit in certain positions, but being uncomfortable can take your focus off the meditation. The most common position for meditation is sitting on the floor with a pillow or sitting on a straight chair. Some people lie in a comfortable position (though you might fall asleep that way).

- ✔ **Close your eyes.** But if you're meditating by focusing on something like a candle flame or flower, you can keep your eyes open.

✔ **Focus on something.** Here are some suggestions:

- **A mantra:** You can repeat a word — such as *God, love,* or *one* — over and over.

- **Your breath:** Focus on the in and out breaths, as well as the space between the breaths.

- **Nothing:** Hold onto nothing. When a thought comes, and it will, let it go. Treat each thought like a passing cloud and keep your mind like an empty blue sky.

But you don't have to be in sitting in a room by yourself with your eyes closed to meditate. You can meditate while taking a walk or otherwise enjoying time outdoors or in a place of worship. Some people meditate with a group or use a meditation tape to help them. Or be in a noisy place and focus on being quiet within yourself. If you're in the "groove," you can do anything in a meditative state — you might call it a state of acute consciousness of the moment.

Guided imagery

If you add mental pictures to your meditation or relaxation, you're engaging in *visualization* or *imagery*. If you use a tape to guide you, that's called *guided imagery*. A guided meditation usually lasts for 20 to 40 minutes; it starts with relaxation of your body and breathing exercises and then brings in images so you can go on an imaginary journey in your mind. For example, you might start on a sandy beach with the sun shining. You can use guided imagery for

✔ **Relaxation:** One benefit of using images is that it helps you relax. If you're thinking about a grassy meadow with wildflowers and butterflies and a soft breeze blowing the fluffy clouds, you're not thinking about your physical or mental problems.

✔ **Healing thoughts:** Some guided meditations include positive healing thoughts. While you're in a relaxed state, you're open to positive suggestion, such as "my body is relaxed," "my liver is healthy," or "my immune system is strong." See Chapter 14 for more examples of positive thoughts to use for healing.

If you can forget your worries and think positive thoughts, you may experience a calming effect and maybe even experience some healing. With guided imagery, you use the images to visualize relaxation and health. To find tapes of guided imagery, ask people at your hep C support group, your mental health or complementary or alternative therapist, or the folks at a bookstore. Some people make their own tapes to listen to.

Chapter 14

Surrounding Yourself with Support

● ●

In This Chapter

▶ Looking at the emotional side of living with hep C

▶ Turning to a support group

▶ Seeing a mental health professional

▶ Networking with others and becoming an advocate

▶ Viewing the glass as half full

● ●

*A*t times, living with a chronic illness can feel overwhelming and devastating. Maybe you're feeling confused, sad, angry, or frustrated at the prospects of facing certain challenges that you'd rather live without.

Whatever feelings and emotions you're experiencing, it helps to know that you're not alone. There are folks out there — both other people with hepatitis C and professionals — who can help you.

And that's the point of this chapter: to suggest some ways to deal with difficult emotions and avoid isolation. So I describe some of the common emotions many people with hepatitis C experience, and then I help you find sources of support, including hep C support groups, mental health professionals, and hepatitis advocacy groups.

But you can also take the task of clearing the gray clouds of negative thoughts, feelings, and emotions into your own hands. So in addition to the self-help suggestions on nutrition, exercise, and relaxation I cover in other chapters, here I describe the process of changing your attitude to look on the bright side. Many people believe that changing how you think can be the most powerful medicine of all.

Handling Your Emotions

You may have mood swings as you live with hep C symptoms such as brain fog or fatigue. Sometimes, you may have feelings of fear, sadness, anger, or depression. Like the weather in London, you may experience every emotion under the sun — including rainstorms, hail, and rainbows — all in a single day! These challenging emotions can come from several sources:

✔ A normal reaction to finding out you have a chronic illness

✔ The hepatitis C virus itself and its effects on your body (see Chapter 4)

✔ Side effects of interferon plus ribavirin treatment (see Chapter 8)

The feelings you get as an emotional reaction to finding out you have hepatitis C may be similar to those of any loss, including denial (no, this isn't really happening), anger (who's to blame for this?), or depression (my life is over). You may also go through stages of bargaining (if I stop smoking, my hep C will disappear) or isolating (I don't want to see anyone).

Like a rainbow that needs both sunshine and rain, ideally, you'll come to a place of some acceptance of the loss of your former health and still see the brightness in your life.

 Keep a record of your feelings. If you have information on the times and days when your emotions go out of whack, that can help you and your healthcare provider figure out a solution. For example, you may find that depression goes hand in hand with fatigue for you. You can then work on increasing your energy (through proper diet and adequate exercise and rest), which in turn can help with depression.

Managing anger

One of the common reactions to getting hepatitis C is anger. For example, if you know how you got hepatitis C, you may be angry at the medical system, your former drug partner, or a former lover. You may be angry at yourself.

 Anger is a normal response to loss, but inappropriate expression of your anger by taking it out on loved ones or yourself can cause more damage. Give safe expression to your anger and then move on. Remaining angry is dangerous because doing so can keep you from getting better. Don't let your resentment poison you.

So you're angry and wondering what you can do about it. Here are some ways to express your anger safely without hurting yourself or anyone else:

- ✔ **Talk it out.** Tell loved ones, friends, and support group members (see the section "Joining Support Groups," later in the chapter) about your feelings.

- ✔ **Punch pillows.** Make sure not to hurt yourself or others when you do this.

- ✔ **Try to cry.** Be specific about why you're crying and angry: "I am so mad at myself for trying drugs. Now look what happened" or "If I had had a decent doctor, maybe I wouldn't have needed that transfusion" or "I hate my ex-husband. I think that so-and-so gave me this disease."

- ✔ **Write down your feelings.** Use a journal to express yourself. You also can use the journal to draw pictures that express your emotions.

- ✔ **Scream!** Just make sure you're alone in a car, out in the desert, or somewhere where you won't scare anyone. Any type of vocalization — from moaning to chanting — can help.

If you find that your anger is escalating or that it doesn't want to stop, see a qualified mental health professional (see the section "Talking with a Mental Health Professional," later in this chapter). Don't take out your anger by hurting yourself or others!

Here are suggestions to help keep your anger at manageable levels:

- ✔ Exercise regularly (see Chapter 13).

- ✔ Practice relaxation (see Chapter 13).

- ✔ Take action. You can harness your energy to do something positive for others (see the section "Taking Action and Networking," later in this chapter).

- ✔ Practice positive thinking (see the section "Staying Positive," later in this chapter).

- ✔ Connect with your spiritual side (see Chapter 13).

Dealing with depression

If you have hepatitis C, feeling blue or sad is a normal response. Depression is a possible side effect of both hepatitis C and interferon treatment. When these feelings won't go away and interfere with your ability to go about your day, you may be suffering from depression. Here are some signs of depression:

- ✔ Persistent sadness
- ✔ Frequent crying
- ✔ Changes in eating or sleeping habits
- ✔ Isolating yourself from friends and family
- ✔ Loss of interest in activities you usually enjoy
- ✔ Difficulty concentrating
- ✔ Feelings of worthlessness
- ✔ Loss of interest in sex
- ✔ Thoughts of death or suicide

If you have any of these symptoms or other concerns about depression, especially if they linger for more than two to four weeks, speak to your hepatitis C doctor, who can help you or refer you to a mental health professional. If you decide to visit a mental health professional before seeing your hepatitis C doctor, make sure to coordinate any use of antidepressants with your hepatitis C doctor.

If you have serious thoughts of death or suicide, call your doctor or 911 immediately.

The following self-help tips may help ease some of the signs of your depression and help alone or in combination with professional counseling or antidepressants:

- ✔ Eat healthy foods (see Chapter 11).
- ✔ Exercise (see Chapter 13).
- ✔ Practice relaxation and proper breathing techniques (see Chapter 13).
- ✔ Meditate and focus on your spirituality (see Chapter 13).
- ✔ Practice positive thinking (see the section "Staying Positive," later in this chapter).
- ✔ Connect with family and friends (see Chapters 15 and 19) and hepatitis C support groups (see the next section, "Joining Support Groups").

Just like exercise helps with fatigue, connecting with others can lift your spirits. Though you might feel like isolating yourself, meeting and connecting with other people, including folks with hepatitis C, may help your feelings of depression.

If some of these tips sound similar to the ones I give to avoid anger, that's no coincidence. Depression and anger are sometimes seen as two sides of the same coin, where depression is anger turned inward.

Some folks on interferon treatment take medication to avoid the well-known and dangerous side effect of depression, which, if untreated, could lead to suicide or relapse of a drug or alcohol addiction. If you've had previous problems with addiction or depression, speak to your doctor before starting treatment. Get your sources of support (medical folks, mental health contacts, family, and friends) lined up before beginning treatment.

Joining Support Groups

Folks who regularly attend support groups say that they're life-savers. The group provides a constant support system through the years of ups and downs associated with living with hepatitis C and treatment. You can discuss your fears and your triumphs with people who understand what you're going through.

Because of the many folks with hepatitis C, support groups have sprung up in many places. In the United States and Canada, more than 350 groups of people with hepatitis C meet to provide mutual support. You can find many more support groups if you count the groups on the Internet.

What you get out of a support group depends on the particular group, the people who attend, and the folks who run the group. Some groups are led by healthcare professionals, such as nurses or social workers; some are led by other people with hep C; and some have medical guest speakers discuss particular topics. But generally, here's what you can expect when you attend a support group:

- ✔ You'll realize that you're not alone.
- ✔ You'll discover how others deal with hep C symptoms, along with other medical, professional, and personal issues.
- ✔ You'll get information about different hepatitis C treatments.
- ✔ You'll make friends who can support you.

At support-group meetings, you'll hear lots of information about hep C from other people. Remember that each of you is different, so discuss any new ideas with your physician before trying them out. An expression popular in 12-step groups (see Chapter 12) works well in this situation: "Take what you like and leave the rest."

Face-to-face support groups

Support groups usually meet once or twice a month in hospitals, libraries, or community centers. If a group meets in a hospital, check ahead, but usually, all are welcome to join, whether or not you have insurance or have a doctor at that hospital.

Some groups are specifically for hepatitis C, while others include hepatitis B, other types of liver disease, or HIV–hepatitis C co-infection. Some groups specialize in pre- and post-liver transplant discussions. Each group has its own policy on whether family and friends can join: Some groups have designated times when family and friends can attend, but otherwise, the groups are closed to non-hep C'ers.

Here are some ways to find a local group:

- ✔ Ask your hepatitis doctor.
- ✔ Call your local hospital or health department, both of which maintain lists of support groups.
- ✔ Call one of the organizations that maintain lists of support groups that I list in Chapter 22.

If you don't find a support group in your area, consider starting one. Here are some issues to consider:

- ✔ **Whom will the group be for?** Only people with hep C? People with other liver diseases? Friends and family of people with hep C?
- ✔ **When and where will you meet?** Try to find a location that's easy to get to and available at a reasonable rate.
- ✔ **What is the format?** Will you have a facilitator or have guest speakers?

Talk to your local hepatologist or gastroenterologist and other healthcare professionals for help getting started. They can put you in contact with other interested professionals and folks with hepatitis C. Also, contact the ALF and HepFI (see Chapter 22 for contact information) for advice on starting a group and listing your group on support-group referral lists.

The Veterans Affairs National Hepatitis C Program has a guide called "Initiating and Maintaining a Hepatitis C Support Group: A How-To Program Guide," which you can find under the educational resources on the program's Web site (www.hepatitis.va.gov).

This hefty 48-page guide can help you start any type of support group, though many suggestions are geared to veterans.

Support groups on the Internet

If you have access to the Internet, you may want to join one of the many different support groups available. When using the Internet for support, consider these pros:

- ✔ Greater anonymity — as long as you don't use your real name or give out personal information

- ✔ Exposure to many more people than you could find in person (especially if you live in a small town)

- ✔ Easier access — you can write and read messages at any time of day or night (if your computer is at home), and you don't have to wait for a monthly meeting

Don't forget these cons about online groups:

- ✔ You won't know anyone's real name or identity. People can — and do — make things up about themselves.

- ✔ The ease of expression on the Internet means that lots gets said, some of which is valuable and true and some of which is harmful and false.

To protect yourself, keep your personal information private and beware any claims for products that are seemingly amazing. Most things that seem too good to be true are just that.

Talking with a Mental Health Professional

Sometimes, emotional or psychological problems become too much to bear alone. You may be having trouble with the medical system, your job, or your family. Talking things over with a qualified mental health professional (such as a social worker, psychologist, or psychiatrist) can steer you toward solutions, including medications, that work for you.

You may need help from a mental health professional in the following situations:

- ✔ You're trying to overcome an addiction to alcohol, drugs, or another substance.

✔ You're suffering from depression.

✔ You're having trouble adjusting to your illness.

✔ You're overwhelmed with feelings of anxiety.

Finding the right therapist or psychiatrist can take a little work. Here are some tips for finding a trained counselor or other professional to help you:

✔ Ask your healthcare professionals for referrals.

✔ Ask other people in your hep C support group for recommendations.

✔ Call your state or local mental health association or associations for psychiatrists or psychologists.

Just as when dealing with any healthcare professional, you also need to consider your health insurance and ability to pay.

Therapy can be short or long term, depending on your needs. Take a moment to think through what's really bothering you. Making a list of the problems that you want to work through can help. Use this list when you check out your potential therapists with a phone call or initial visit to see whether you're compatible. You may want to ask whether the therapist has worked with people with hepatitis C. If you have strong feelings about different types of treatment, bring that topic up. See what kind of vibes you get from the therapist. You need to feel comfortable with this person so you can trust him or her with your personal feelings and problems.

Finding a mental health professional to help you may take some work, but getting the personal support you need is worth the effort.

Taking Action and Networking

A great way to channel your energy and help others is to do some hepatitis C advocacy work. You can network with other people with hep C and at the same time take the following actions:

✔ Educate the public and professionals about hepatitis C transmission.

✔ Ask the government to provide additional funding for research.

✔ Advocate for more hepatitis C screening programs.

✔ Advocate for prevention and harm-reduction programs.

✔ Help the uninsured and working poor get treatment.

See Chapter 22 for a starting point for agencies and organizations that use volunteers. Many people with hepatitis C also use the Internet for advocacy and networking. You can find a huge number of Web sites devoted to hepatitis C, many of which are organized by people with hepatitis C. If you have computer or writing skills, you can help out with a site that's up and running or create your own site where you can spread your message.

Staying Positive

The body, mind, and emotions are interconnected. If you're emotionally off balance, that could be due to hep C's effect on your body and your thoughts. (I also discuss the mind-body connection in Chapter 13 while discussing stress.) Because the power of your thoughts is so strong, positive thinking can help you feel better.

A positive attitude lies behind positive thinking. You sometimes have to "make believe" that you have a positive attitude until your mind catches up on its own. Here's how you'll benefit from this positive attitude:

✔ You'll feel better emotionally, spiritually, and physically.

✔ You'll be more pleasant to those around you, including family, friends, co-workers, medical office employees, and even supermarket cashiers. And they'll be nicer to you in return!

Because the mind and body are connected, changing your attitude to a positive one may help your immune system and liver (see Chapter 13).

Like any habit, positive thinking can be learned. The goal is to substitute positive thoughts for negative thoughts. Making the change can be challenging at first. Modern life supports negative thoughts. Many newspapers and television shows give heavy coverage to reports of crime, violence, hate, and war. Finding reports of compassion, healing, resolution, and love can be harder. But you can do it. Here are some suggestions for changing your thinking:

✔ **Look for the positive.** When I'm feeling negative while I'm out walking, I make myself count ten nice things around me. See whether that idea works for you. You may not feel positive if you're dealing with hepatitis C problems, but try to find something positive anyway.

✔ **Make a gratitude list.** You can keep a separate notebook for things you're thankful for and write your list each night. Or you can simply make mental notes of what you're grateful for.

After you start your list, you'll be amazed at all the things to appreciate in your life.

✔ **Pay attention to your thoughts.** During meditation or quiet times, you can "hear" the thoughts running through your head. Do your thoughts make you feel good or bad? Noticing your negative thoughts helps in the process of letting them go.

✔ **Use positive affirmations.** You may need to consciously think positive thoughts at first to add them to your thinking repertoire. Some people write them down, meditate on them, or use tapes of affirmations. To affirm is to say yes, and an affirmation is a thought that says, "yes, it's possible." An affirmation is a positive thought. So instead of letting negative comments or thoughts, such as "Life stinks," run through your mind or come out of your mouth, try focusing on a positive affirmation, such as "Each day is a precious gift."

Affirmations are most useful when you either create your own or pick the ones that resonate with you.

Try writing down your own negative thoughts. Then counter them with positive alternatives. Here are some examples:

Negative Thought	Positive Alternative
I will always be sick.	My body is perfect and whole.
My liver is ruined.	My liver is healing.
This virus has got me beat.	I know my immune system is clearing hep C from my body.
I'll never work again.	I'm looking forward to finding new ways to work.
I'll die before I get a new liver.	A new liver is on its way to me.

Write your positive thoughts or affirmations in a way that's comfortable for you. You can keep them in your hep C notebook, along with all your test results and doctors' notes, to remind you to look on the bright side — no matter what. As one wise woman said to me, "My attitude is all I can change, and that's about 90 percent of everything."

Try focusing on the present. Thinking about the future can bring worry and fear, which isn't useful when it clouds the appreciation of today. Make the choice to enjoy today, and know that you'll deal with the future when it comes. If you enjoy today, you're more likely to enjoy tomorrow.

Chapter 15

Working through Relationships and Telling Others

....

In This Chapter

▶ Figuring out whom to tell about your hep C

▶ Getting prepared to tell others

▶ Discussing sex with your partner

▶ Telling your children

▶ Coping with the stigma

....

*T*elling the people whom you care about and love that you have hepatitis C can be trying and difficult at times, but you can do it, and I'm here to help make the process easier. Telling others about your health is important. You need their support to deal with your illness and treatment. And they need to take measures to protect themselves from getting infected. But you have the choice of whom you want to tell and when, why, and how you want to tell them.

Your first step is to prepare yourself with information on transmission and disease progression (which I discuss in Chapters 2 and 4, respectively) so that you can answer any questions that come up. Then you need to decide whom to tell about your hep C. I don't want to sugarcoat this matter: Some people may react with fear or discrimination. To minimize the possibility of encountering this type of closed-minded attitude, make sure to think ahead before telling people outside your closest family members.

In this chapter, I help you decide whom to tell, how to prepare for the conversation, and when and how to do it. I also help you plan for the most intimate of conversations — whether you're married or single, telling your sexual partner about your hep C is the responsible thing to do — and offer some tips for dealing with your sex life. Finally, I spend time on communicating with your children about your illness.

Deciding Whom to Tell

Whom you decide to tell about your hepatitis C is completely up to you. The advantage of telling people is that you may get their support. The disadvantage is that you may have to deal with their fears or discrimination toward you.

Take a bit of time to consider whom you wish to tell, including the following:

- ✔ Your children
- ✔ Your parents
- ✔ Friends and other family
- ✔ People at work

Partners and household members

 You might tell your partner or spouse first. She's likely the person that you feel closest to and most comfortable with, plus she's likely to be a primary source of support. But you'll probably *both* be upset at first until you have time to digest the news. Your loved one will probably be concerned about you and about herself as she wonders if she was infected, too. So give it time.

 Consider that household members or sex partners will want to know. They care about you and are potentially at risk if they have shared a household item (a razor or toothbrush, for example) or have sex with you. Read about how hepatitis C is transmitted in Chapter 2.

Any member of your household — spouse, partner, or child — may eventually find out if you become ill with hep C or while you're undergoing treatment. So you may want to tell them at a time when everyone is relatively calm and you're not in a crisis of ill health.

You have the choice of deciding when to tell everyone on a case-by-case basis. You may want to wait until you're feeling strong enough to handle your loved ones' reactions. On the other hand, don't wait too long, because you need their support and help.

If you want your personal information kept private, you can ask the person to keep the information confidential. Ideally, your close friends and family will respect your wishes. Asking children to keep secrets is more difficult, however, and doing so may not be the best thing for the child. When you tell people, you need to be prepared for the fact that they may tell other people.

People at work

I don't recommend that you tell anyone in the workplace until you have carefully thought through the ramifications of how daily workplace interactions and your future employment with the company will be affected. Consult your doctor, legal advisor, and family members before deciding whom should know about your hepatitis C, when to tell them, or even whether to tell them.

You may wonder why you have to be so careful. The combination of people's prejudice against an infectious disease such as hepatitis C and your potential inability to perform your job could lead to sticky social and legal issues. Some people at work may stigmatize you and make your life miserable (see the section "Dealing with Stigma," later in this chapter).

Before you tell anyone on the job, discuss your situation with a lawyer or disability office (state or federal). Unfortunately, the Americans with Disabilities Act (www.ada.gov) has only a limited ability to protect you against discrimination (see Chapter 16 for a discussion of work and financial issues).

Folks exposed to your blood

You should consider telling two categories of people about your hep C. In most cases, you are not legally obliged to tell the following people, so it's up to you:

> ✓ **People with whom you shared injected drugs with in the past:** You may save their lives by letting them know that they may be infected with hep C and should get tested. If they find out early enough, they can get treated and prevent development of end-stage liver disease or liver cancer.

✔ **People who are in contact with your blood now:** These people should always take proper precautions to protect themselves, but you can let them know so they can be absolutely careful:

- Dentists, nurses, and other healthcare workers
- Acupuncturists
- Tattoo artists or body piercers
- Sex partners (in some cases; see Chapter 2)

Preparing to Tell Others

After you decide whom you want to tell about your hepatitis C and when, take the time to prepare for the conversation. Arm yourself with information about the disease of hepatitis and how it spreads by exposure to blood. And if you're approaching someone who may be particularly difficult to tell (your mother, for example), you may want to bring along a supportive person (your spouse or sister, for example).

Here are some steps that may make telling others about your condition a little easier:

1. **Prepare yourself emotionally.**

   Get emotional support for yourself so that you're prepared for the conversation. Hepatitis C support groups or mental health professionals can help (see Chapter 14).

2. **Get the facts about transmission and the disease and collect information to share with the other person.**

   Speak to your doctor and get advice from her. Read through this book and other information so you can answer questions. And have something on hand (like this book or shorter pamphlets, fact sheets, and so on) for the person (such as an adult or older child) to read.

3. **Practice what you'll say beforehand, keeping in mind that being clear and honest is the best approach.**

   I have the hepatitis C virus. Hepatitis C is a bloodborne virus.

   This step is especially helpful when you're going to talk with children or if you're feeling a little shaky.

4. **Be prepared for questions that people might ask, including the following:**

How did *you* get this virus? Here are some suggested answers:

> *I once used a shared needle to try some drugs, a long time ago.*
>
> *I had a blood transfusion during an operation or after my car accident.*
>
> *I'm not sure. It could be from my tattoo or from being in the army.*

What will happen to you? Are you sick now? Consider these possible responses:

> *I don't have any symptoms, but my doctor found it through a blood test. I have to keep up my testing. But I feel fine.*
>
> *I've changed my diet, and I'm exercising every day so I can stay healthy. I know I can beat this virus.*
>
> *I've started treatment, and I'm not feeling too good because of the side effects.*
>
> *I didn't know I had hepatitis C until I went to the hospital and found out I have cirrhosis. I'm scared, but I know I have a good doctor who's helping me.*

Did I catch it from you? Here's what you can tell your friend:

> *You can get tested, if you want. But it's not so easy to catch unless you were exposed to my blood. The virus is transmitted through blood.*

Can I catch it from you? You can answer this way:

> *You can't get hep C through kissing or eating from the same plate or hugging.*
>
> *You'll be fine as long as you don't use my toothbrush or razor, because there might be some blood on it.*

5. **Be prepared to give the person time to process the information.**

   Your friend or relative may be confused or shocked after hearing about your hep C. Reassure the person that you're taking care of yourself. You may want to call or visit the person in a week or so to follow up.

After you tell trusted friends and family members about your illness, they may ask you how they can help and support you. Think about what help you might need now or in the future (see Chapter 19 for ways friends and family can help), and keep their names and phone numbers in your hep C notebook, which I discuss in more detail in Chapter 5.

Talking about Sex and Dating

Hepatitis C is called a sexually transmitted disease because it *can* be transmitted that way. However, it's not usually transmitted through sex. Here are the official recommendations about preventing the spread of hep C through sex:

- ✔ If you're in a monogamous, long-term heterosexual relationship, you have a very low risk of spreading hepatitis C. Discuss the matter with your partner and doctor.

- ✔ If you have multiple sex partners or sex that involves blood, you're at higher risk of spreading hep C that way. You're advised to practice safer sex, which I discuss in Chapter 2.

- ✔ If you are a man and have sex with other men, consider your sex practices and their risks. Use a latex condom for anal sex and take precautions against getting hepatitis A, which is spread through contact with feces (see Chapter 2).

If you're married or in a partnership

Have an open discussion with your sex partner about sexual transmission of hepatitis C. The two of you can bring any concerns to your healthcare provider. You can decide whether you wish to use condoms or make any other changes in your sex life to reduce the possibility of exposure to blood (see Chapter 2).

Your partner may wish to also get tested for hepatitis C, which can allay fears about transmission. To discuss problems about lack of interest in sex or performance issues, see "Dealing with sexual problems," later in this chapter.

When you're single

Having a diagnosis of hepatitis C can feel scary, especially if you're single. You may feel that you'll never have a partner or make love again. But consider that in the United States alone, nearly 4 million people have been infected with hep C, some of whom, like you, are single. Other people with long-term illnesses manage to find love.

You're more than your disease. You're still the person you were before hep C who needs to have relationships and a social life. Even if you don't have lots of energy or complete physical health, you are still lovable. Keep your social life active with platonic and romantic relationships. Here are some tips:

✔ Think positively and try to find a partner or friends (with or without hepatitis C) worthy of you. If someone is fearful or disrespectful of your hepatitis C, letting them go is probably the best solution.

✔ Go to hepatitis C events and support groups to meet others with hepatitis C.

✔ Consider looking into some dating lists on the Web that are specifically for people with hepatitis C. Be careful, however, not to divulge personal information on the Web, which I mention in Chapter 14 in a discussion of online support groups for hepatitis C. If you plan to meet someone in person whom you've found through the Web, follow safety practices outlined in books such as *Online Dating For Dummies,* by Judith Silverstein, MD, and Michael Lasky, JD (Wiley).

At some point, before you become sexually involved with a new partner, you need to tell the person about your hepatitis C and also discuss protection against other sexually transmitted diseases (see the section "Preparing to Tell Others," earlier in this chapter).

Dealing with sexual problems

You may have a lowered sexual desire (decreased libido) or difficulties performing sexually. For a man, this problem can be impotence or ejaculation problems; a woman may have an inability to achieve an orgasm. Sexual problems can arise from the effects of hepatitis C virus or drug treatment on your mind and body. You may have fatigue or depression, both of which decrease interest in sex.

It's important to talk to your partner about your concerns. You deserve to have loving connections, even when you may not be up to your normal sexual activities.

Examining some causes

Whether you're straight or gay, married or single, young or old, male or female, hep C can result in a loss of interest in sex, adding to your stress. Here are some reasons your libido, or interest in sex, may wane:

✔ Liver disease may affect male and female sex hormones (which I discuss in Chapter 18).

✔ The symptoms of hep C, mainly fatigue but also feelings of nausea or headaches, are definitely enough to put you out of the mood.

✔ Treatment with combination interferon therapy has another set of side effects that lessen your desire for sex.

✔ Loss of interest in sex is a common side effect of depression, which is common with hep C *and* interferon treatment (see Chapter 14 for more on depression).

✔ Side effects of many antidepressants include loss of interest in sex, inability to have an orgasm, and/or loss of erection.

✔ Worry about sexual transmission of hep C can dampen the mood.

Because sexual problems can result from so many different reasons, talk to your physician about specific help for your particular situation. You may be able to change medications if that's causing the problem. Your doctor can prescribe a medication to help men with erection problems. Hormone-based vaginal creams may help women.

Talking with your partner

How do you discuss this topic with your loved one? Your partner may take your disinterest as rejection, so let your spouse know that the problem is not with him or your relationship but with your health. Keep the lines of communication open and be honest.

1. **State clearly how you feel:**

   I love you so much. I want to make love. I know it's been a while.

2. **State your situation or problem:**

   I'm just too tired/anxious/sick. The medications have taken away my physical desire.

3. **State what you can do:**

   Can we cuddle? I'll speak to the doctor about this. How about on the weekend, when I have more energy?

State your situation truthfully but kindly and don't make promises you can't keep.

Communicating with Children

Being prepared before telling your children is especially important. If you have symptoms or side effects, your children will probably know about it. Children usually are perceptive enough to realize what's going on in a household.

Tell your children about the disease of hepatitis C. The older the children are or the more children want to know about the disease, the more you can tell them. Give them a brief summary of what they can expect about your symptoms or energy levels. (In Chapter 17, I cover the unique aspects facing children with hepatitis C. Check it out for additional tips on how to explain hep C to kids.)

Tell your children that you're doing everything you can to get well, including taking naps, seeing the doctor, eating healthy food, and taking medicines. Children need to be assured of the following:

- ✔ That you love them.

- ✔ That you plan to be around for a long time.

- ✔ That someone will always be available to take care of them, if you can't.

- ✔ That they did not give you the disease.

- ✔ That they can't catch it. Here's your opportunity to explain how hepatitis C is caught (and that everyone will be sure to use his or her own toothbrush and razor) and how it's *not* caught (through the air, by kissing, by eating together, and so on). See Chapter 2 for more information on protecting others.

Your children may respond by offering to help, which is excellent for you (especially if you tire easily) and them! Give them chores that are appropriate for their age.

Dealing with Stigma

Some people in the general public, or even in your family or workplace, aren't educated about the nature of hep C (see the sidebar "Hep C S.M.A.R.T." in this chapter). As a result, they may view your disease as a stigma — a mark of shame or disgrace associated with the virus. People who consider hep C as a type of stigma may

- ✔ Treat you as contaminated or unclean because you have hep C, which is an infectious disease.

- ✔ Assume that you're a drug addict (and many people have negative views of drug addicts).

Because of the stigma sometimes attached to hep C, you may fear that people will treat you differently, leave you, deny you health or life insurance, or fire you from your job. You may even fear violence if one of your family members or sex partners is worried that you have infected them.

Hep C S.M.A.R.T.

The American Gastroenterological Association (AGA) carried out a study with Harris Interactive (of the famous Harris poll) to look at attitudes about hepatitis C. The survey questioned people not infected with hep C, people infected with hep C, and physicians (primary care physicians and specialists).

This study was part of an AGA program called "Be Hep C S.M.A.R.T (Shattering Myths and Reinforcing Truths)," designed to educate both the public and health-care providers about hep C transmission, diagnosis, and treatment. Here are some study findings:

✔ Some general confusion exists in the general public about hep C transmission. For example, 32 percent of uninfected people questioned thought that hep C was transmitted by contaminated water or food. Forty-two percent didn't know that contact was through exposure to infected blood.

✔ Stigma is clearly a concern of people with hep C. Seventy-four percent of people with hepatitis C believed the public thinks that the virus infects mainly drug addicts and people with unhealthy lifestyles. Interestingly, only 30 percent of the general public without hepatitis C believed this. Only 12 percent of the general public believed that they couldn't get a disease like hep C.

If you're informed about hepatitis C and have a support group — including healthcare professionals, friends, family, and others with hepatitis C — you'll be much more likely to find ways to deal with any discrimination or rejection that comes your way.

Chapter 16

Facing Financial and Workplace Challenges

● ●

In This Chapter

▶ Staying on the job with hepatitis C

▶ Understanding your health insurance

▶ Getting help when you quit working

▶ Planning for financial security

● ●

*L*iving with a chronic illness like hepatitis C affects your employment and financial life. Your costs of living may increase at the same time that your earning potential decreases if you have medical expenses and need to take some time off work or work reduced hours. Either the symptoms of hepatitis C or the side effects of medical treatment (or both) can make it difficult or impossible to continue working.

When it comes to work and finances, think things through in advance so that you're prepared for the future. Get professional advice from a lawyer, benefits advisor, or financial planner to help you make decisions that can affect your future healthcare and the finances of your family.

Keep all your records! Make copies of every letter or form you send in regard to the financial and insurance-related aspects of your healthcare, and keep every letter you receive. When you have a phone conversation with someone about benefits or insurance, keep notes of the conversation, including the date, time, and name of the person you speak with. Being organized — or even superorganized! — helps when you need to file a claim or complaint.

In this chapter, I present information on work issues, health insurance, financial planning, and applying for disability when you have hepatitis C.

Working with Hepatitis C

For most people with hep C, the goal is to continue working as long as possible. Working provides:

✔ Income and benefits (medical/dental/vision insurance, disability insurance, life insurance, and a pension plan) for you and your family

✔ A way to express your skills and talents

✔ A connection to the larger community

If your ability to work is impaired by hep C, this can affect your financial status and your self-esteem. How hep C affects your work life depends on what type of symptoms you have and how they affect your ability to perform your job.

If you have no noticeable effects of the virus at this time, you don't have a reason to tell anyone at work about your hep C. You may not develop symptoms that affect your ability to work for many years. But now is a good time to collect all the information on your health insurance and other benefits so that you have it if the need arises.

Dealing with symptoms on the job

Hepatitis C can trigger debilitating symptoms (see Chapter 4), and treatment with interferon (see Chapter 8) can add its own list of side effects. You can have a range of symptoms that can affect your ability to work.

Most people with hepatitis C don't develop the most serious complications but may suffer from symptoms such as fatigue or brain fog that can challenge your ability to work well. See the self-help tips to deal with fatigue later in this section and also check out Chapter 13.

Keep a list of symptoms in your hep C notebook (which I explain in detail in Chapter 5). A running diary of your symptoms helps you find any patterns. If you need to apply for disability insurance (see the section "Looking at Disability Benefits," later in the chapter), this information is essential.

When you observe your symptoms and note how they affect your ability to work, you'll find that your symptoms fall into one of these categories:

✔ **Short term or temporary:** With short-term symptoms, you may need to take a temporary leave of absence, reduce your hours, or avoid certain procedures at your job (heavy lifting for example) for a short period of time (less than a year) in the following situations:

- You're going through a brief rough patch.

- You're on interferon treatment, and your symptoms will get better when that's over.

- You're on an alternative treatment that will eventually help your symptoms.

✔ **Long term or permanent:** Consider leaving your job and applying for disability insurance when

- You've had difficult symptoms for years.

- Your disease has progressed or presented itself to you as late-stage cirrhosis.

These categories aren't hard and fast. Medical treatment or the body's own defenses can help a so-called long-term or permanent condition improve. The major issue for most people when contemplating leaving work is how they'll support themselves and their families. The United States (and many other countries) offers national support in the form of disability benefits for folks who are unable to work because of chronic illness. I discuss short-term and long-term disability benefits in the United States in the section "Looking at Disability Benefits," later in this chapter.

Fatigue is a symptom of both hep C and a side effect of interferon treatment. (Chapter 13 has more about fatigue.) Needless to say, experiencing fatigue can make the workday difficult. But healthy eating and other lifestyle changes can help you maintain energy at work:

✔ Eat small frequent healthy meals/snacks (see Chapter 11).

✔ Avoid sugary, fatty foods (see Chapter 11).

✔ Practice deep-breathing exercises (see Chapter 13).

✔ Get fresh air and go out into the sunlight to rejuvenate yourself at work. Walk around the block.

Your healthcare practitioner can help you sort through your symptoms and help you decide when to make changes in your work life or even if you should stop working and apply for disability. Your doctor is an important ally because he can write letters attesting to your medical condition for work or Social Security purposes.

Telling your boss and making changes

Sometimes, despite your best efforts, you'll have to make some changes at work. If your symptoms become severe enough to interfere with your work, you may need to talk to your employer about taking some time off or changing your hours. Put off telling your employer about your illness until you've carefully considered potential problems. Many workplaces have antidiscrimination policies, but you may run into problems in some workplaces and with certain co-workers (if you also confide in them). If possible, get professional advice (from an employment or disability expert).

When you're ready to talk to your boss about hepatitis C, follow these suggestions:

- ✔ Choose a time when you and your boss have some privacy.

- ✔ Bring this book or other materials to leave with your boss, if she wants further information.

- ✔ Emphasize that you're treating the disease and its side effects and *you're not contagious or a danger to anyone.*

If you experience discrimination on the job or you're fired after discussing the issue with your employer, you may be able to get help through the Americans with Disabilities Act, described in the section "Getting your federal acts together," later in this chapter.

Some folks need to change the type of work they do. Perhaps you're just too tired to continue your job that requires physical labor in the hot sun. Or you've temporarily lost the ability to focus on your job. You may be able to negotiate options to help you keep your job:

- ✔ Working part-time

- ✔ Changing some of your tasks

- ✔ Working from home

If you decide to work part-time, check first to make sure that you don't lose your health insurance and other benefits.

Researching Health Insurance

Directly paying doctor and hospital fees that range from thousands to tens of thousands of dollars per year isn't an option for most people. Instead, you may have insurance through your job or your spouse's job, as a veteran (through the Veterans Administration), as a senior citizen (through Medicare), or as a person with a low income (through Medicaid). Or you may be one of the millions of Americans without health insurance.

In addition to the resources listed throughout this chapter, HCV Advocate has a large number of articles dealing with benefits, insurance, and financial issues for people with hep C on its Web site, www.hcvadvocate.org/hepatitis/living_w_ hepatitis_C.asp#2.

Another resource for information on hepatitis C and health insurance is the Web site www.hepatitisneighborhood.com, which has a section called "Financing Your Care" that links to useful articles. You must sign up (for free) to use the site, provided by Priority Healthcare.

Getting a handle on the basics

In the United States today, health plans vary widely, although most are a type of a managed care plan (such as a health maintenance organization, or HMO). I give you some definitions of common terms that give you a handle on the ins and outs of health insurance. Use them to figure out what type of policy you have, what it covers, and what it doesn't.

What type of plan do you have?

The name of your plan can help you identify the benefits you have. Read the small print to get the details of your particular plan.

- ✔ **Fee for service (indemnity):** In this more expensive type of plan, you or the healthcare providers are reimbursed for the amount paid. You can choose which physician to see and when to see them. You usually have a yearly deductible and frequently pay a percentage of the cost of each medical visit.

- ✔ **Managed care:** These types of health plans aim to control rising costs of healthcare by limiting which doctors you can visit and what types of treatments are covered.

- ✔ **Health maintenance organization (HMO):** In this form of pre-paid health insurance, you pay a fixed *premium* (money paid for the health insurance policy). The HMO pays certain doctors to provide this healthcare, and the physicians are called *in-network*.

✔ **Point of service (POS) plan and preferred provider organization (PPO):** These plans fall in between a managed plan and an indemnity plan. You can see doctors out of network, but doing so will cost you more. Each insurer has its own definitions for these policies and how much more you pay to see out-of-network providers.

Your employer may also offer you a healthcare savings account called MSA (medical savings account) or FSA (flexible spending account).

How about government health plans?

The Centers for Medicare and Medicaid Services (CMS) is an agency within the U.S. Department of Health and Human Services. Programs for which CMS is responsible include Medicare, Medicaid, and State Children's Health Insurance Program (SCHIP). Here's some info on those programs:

✔ **Medicaid:** The federal and state health insurance program for Americans with low incomes. Every state has different rules, and you may have a small co-payment for some services. Contact your state office for more information. If you aren't a citizen of the United States but are a U.S. resident, you may be eligible for benefits under certain circumstances. For more information, see www.cms.hhs.gov/medicaid.

✔ **Medicare:** The federal health insurance program for people aged 65 or older, people who have permanent kidney failure, and some people under age 65 with disabilities. Coverage includes the following:

  • **Hospital insurance:** Provides for treatment while at a hospital or while receiving some types of home or hospice care. This part of Medicare (Part A) is available to all persons age 65 or over as part of Social Security.

  • **Medical insurance:** Covers physician and other outpatient services. You may pay a premium for this elective coverage (known as Part B).

  To contact Medicare, visit the Web site www.medicare.gov or call 800-MEDICARE (800-633-4227).

✔ **SCHIP:** This program helps uninsured children from low-income families who don't qualify for Medicaid.

For more information on any of these programs, visit www.cms.hhs.gov.

Who's in charge?

You may see more than one type of doctor if you have hep C. A *primary care physician* (PCP) is your healthcare gatekeeper and refers you to specialists, such as gastroenterologists, or for specific tests. (See Chapter 5 to read more about PCPs and specialists who treat hepatitis C.) Generally, a managed care plan requires that your PCP refer you to a specialist. In a fee-for-service plan, you don't need a referral, and you can decide whom you wish to visit.

What are your out-of-pocket costs?

As a patient, you usually pay some of your healthcare costs. A *premium* is the regular amount (usually monthly) you pay toward your healthcare insurance; that amount usually comes directly out of your paycheck.

Co-insurance or *co-pay* is an additional amount of money that you pay for certain services. For example, in an 80/20 split, the insurance company pays 80 percent of the cost, and you pay 20 percent of the cost. Another example is the $15 co-pay you may be charged at each office visit.

A *deductible* is the amount you must pay, each calendar year or other period, toward approved medical care before your insurance company will start to pay your medical bills.

What's covered and what's not?

You need to know what things your particular health plan will pay for because plans vary widely. An HMO has a list of doctors and test facilities it has negotiated to work with. These doctors and facilities are *in-network* providers. If you go to an *out-of-network* doctor or facility that's not on the approved list, you may pay extra.

Exclusions are health conditions or procedures not covered by your policy. Frequently, pregnancy and childbirth are in this category.

Precertification means that certain procedures, doctor or hospital visits, and medications may need prior approval from your insurance company; otherwise, insurance won't cover them. If you don't get precertification and insurance is denied, you may have to pay out of pocket and then pursue reimbursement with your company.

Preventive care or *preventive medicine,* also called a check-up or routine physical, refers to tests and office visits that look for illness before you have any symptoms or complaints. Preventive care includes things like blood tests, mammograms, prostate exams, and EKGs (electrocardiograms). Managed care plans are more likely to cover these costs than indemnity plans.

Filling up on prescription facts

You may be taking combination peginterferon plus ribavirin medication (see Chapter 8) or taking other drugs as prescribed by your doctor. These prescription drugs can be very costly and may or not be included or excluded from your health plan. Prescription drugs fall into one of these categories:

- ✔ **Brand name:** When drugs are first marketed, they're sold by the company that has a patent to be the sole producer of the drug for a period of time.

- ✔ **Generic:** After the patent expires, drugs may be produced by other companies for a lower cost. Your doctor and/or insurance company may not allow or approve of generic drugs.

When you begin any new drug (or change health insurance policies) check to make sure that your drugs will be covered.

Making a complaint

You are your best advocate when making sure that you get the best healthcare possible. If you want to visit a certain specialist, take a certain medication, or have a certain procedure that isn't covered by your health plan, take action:

- ✔ Speak to your doctor to see if she'll write a letter for you.

- ✔ Call your insurance company and ask about the procedure for lodging a complaint.

- ✔ Write to your insurance company and make a case for what you want. For example, explain that no other liver specialist is on your health plan within a 50-mile radius.

Keep copies of all correspondence from your insurance company, document any telephone calls, and print out all e-mails. Follow up your case and don't be surprised if you get what you need!

Living without health insurance in the United States

A snapshot picture by the U.S. Census Bureau of health insurance coverage in the United States in 2003 reveals that 84.4 percent of Americans have health insurance and 15.6 percent — or 45 million people — do not. What can you do if you are uninsured and need healthcare? Here are some suggestions:

✔ See whether you can receive care from local or state agencies, such as the Medicaid program (see the "How about government health plans?" section, earlier in the chapter).

✔ The drug companies that make treatments for hepatitis C offer compensation for people without health insurance. I include the companies' telephone numbers in Chapter 22.

✔ Some clinics offer testing for hepatitis C (Chapter 6) and advice for further treatment.

✔ If you need a liver transplant and don't have health insurance, you may qualify for help (see Chapter 9).

✔ Agencies that offer assistance to people with hepatitis may be able to direct you to more info and help (see Chapter 22).

Getting compensation for hepatitis C

In some cases, the governments of Canada and the United Kingdom (UK) are providing financial compensation for individuals (and families) who were infected by hepatitis C as a result of a transfusion blood product.

In Canada, a class-action suit is being filed for people infected through contaminated blood between January 1, 1986, and July 1, 1990. You can get information by contacting Administrator of the Hepatitis C Claims Centre, P.O. Box 2370, Station D, Ottawa, Ontario, K1P 5W5; phone 877-434-0944; Web site www.hepc8690.com. If you were infected before January 1, 1986, and after July 1, 1990, or you want links to province-specific compensation, check out the compensation section of the Web site of the Hepatitis C Society of Canada, www.hepatitiscsociety.com/english/HepCCompensation.htm.

In the UK, the government pays if you received blood or blood products from the National Health Service (NHS) before 1991, when screening was started. This plan is called *ex-gratia,* which means that the government will pay you but not admit liability. The payment is _20,000 pounds if you have hepatitis C and a further 25,000 pounds if your disease is more advanced (you have cirrhosis, liver cancer, or liver transplant). This fund became active in July 2004.

For more information, contact the Skipton Fund, P.O. Box 50107, London, SW1H 0YF, UK; phone 020-7233-0057; e-mail apply@skiptonfund.org, Web site www.skiptonfund.org.

Although no amount of money truly compensates for the loss of health, well-being, or life, I applaud the fact that some health services are acknowledging their role in the transmission of the hepatitis C virus. Acknowledgment must also go to the hard work of some people with hepatitis C and their lawyers and friends who fought to bring about compensation benefits.

Nationalized health insurance

Health insurance in countries with national health plans (such as the United Kingdom, Canada, and Australia) generally provides healthcare for all residents, regardless of the ability to pay. At the same time, the system allows for private payment or private insurance that results in a somewhat two-tiered system: those on the national plan and those who also have a private plan. One advantage of a nationalized plan, in addition to not having to pay for most services, is that the paperwork load for the patient is vastly reduced.

Whatever the advantages and disadvantages of healthcare systems between or within different countries, it pays to find out as much as you can about your healthcare insurance.

Looking at Disability Benefits

For some folks, a time comes when they can't work like they used to. The onset of serious symptoms that lead to an inability to work *(disability)* may come a long time after the initial diagnosis with hepatitis C. You may have short-term or long-term symptoms, which translate into a short-term or long-term disability.

Defining types of benefits

If you become unable to work, you may need financial assistance. You may qualify for employer and state benefits, and it's up to you to find out what benefits you can apply for. Speak to your human resources/benefits office (if you have one) or your employer, do some research in your local library, or use the telephone book to find information for your state offices. (I list the contact details for Social Security in the "Applying for government disability insurance" section later in the chapter.) The type of benefit you need depends on how long you'll need assistance.

Short-term disability (STD)

This period can last up to one year. Depending on how long you're ill and your particular benefits at your job, you may be able to use your sick leave for a short-term illness. Other benefits to look into include employer or state benefits or the Family and Medical Leave Act (see the section of the same name later in the chapter).

Long-term disability (LTD)

This coverage takes over after short-term disability. At this point, you can also apply for state disability and Social Security disability (see the "Applying for government disability insurance" section, later in the chapter).

If you're on long-term disability, you must reapply for benefits at regular intervals to prove that you remain unable to work. Long-term disability lasts until you qualify for Medicare, at retirement age, or 24 months after you've been on Social Security disability.

Getting your federal acts together

To prevent discrimination and also to protect workers who have medical needs, two federal laws were enacted in the United States.

Americans with Disabilities Act

The Americans with Disabilities Act (ADA) protects you against discrimination on the job, but it applies only if your employer knows that you have hepatitis C. If you haven't told your employer about your hepatitis C, you can't make a complaint about discrimination due to your hepatitis C.

Generally, this law covers employers with more than 15 employees. The ADA defines *disability* as a physical or mental impairment that substantially limits at least one major life activity. People who are discriminated against because of their known association with a person with a disability are also protected by the ADA. The ADA covers other types of discrimination, ranging from transportation to education to healthcare. To find out more about this act, visit the ADA Web site at www.usdoj.gov/crt/ada or call 800-514-0301.

Family and Medical Leave Act

According to the Family and Medical Leave Act (FMLA), eligible employees of certain firms or organizations (with more than 50 employees) are entitled to a 12-week unpaid leave every 12 months for valid medical or family reasons. Serious medical conditions or treatments are covered under the FMLA. While you are on FMLA, your health benefits are retained, and generally, your job will be held for you. Read more at www.dol.gov/esa/whd/fmla or call 866-4-USA-DOL (866-487-2365).

Applying for government disability insurance

If you're unable to work due to your hepatitis C, you may be eligible for United States government disability benefits (SSDI and SSI), administered by the Social Security Administration. Your disability must be long term; Social Security does not give short-term insurance. The two government benefits you can apply for are the following:

- **Social Security Disability Insurance (SSDI):** You may qualify if you've paid into this insurance through your prior employment.

- **Supplemental Security Income (SSI):** This benefit is based on financial need.

Getting a head start on the disability application

Here's a place to start the information-gathering and -organizing process when applying for Social Security disability insurance. This information comes from the "Medical and Job Worksheet - Adult" from the Disability Starter Kit that is used to prepare for an interview or to complete the Disability Report. Here is some of the info you'll need to provide:

- The date (month, date, and year) you became unable to work.

- The medical condition(s) that keep you from working.

- Each healthcare practitioner who has treated your condition. For each one, gather the healthcare practitioner's name, address, and phone number; your patient ID number with that practitioner; and the dates (month and year) of your visit(s).

- Visits to hospitals or clinics. Include the name, address, phone number, and hospital/clinic number (see your paperwork or call the hospital) and the date (month and year) of each visit.

- Your medications. Include the name of the medication, why you take it, and the name of the doctor who prescribed it.

- All medical tests you have taken or are scheduled to take. Include the name of the test, the location of the test, the name of the doctor who ordered the test, and the date of the test.

- Your medical assistance number. If you're already receiving state Medicaid benefits, check your card for that number.

- Your jobs for the past 15 years. Include your job titles, the types of businesses where you worked, and the dates worked (month and year).

To get more information, go to the Web site www.socialsecurity.gov/disability/ and click on the Disability Starter Kits link; call 800-772-1213; or go to your local Social Security office.

Social Security determines whether you fit its definition of disabled by asking a series of questions. You must demonstrate that your illness is severe enough to keep you from working at your previous job or any other job. You must also not make more than a specified amount, which at the time of this writing is $810 per year.

You can apply for disability benefits by going online at www. ssa.gov, visiting your local Social Security office (check your phone book for the location), or calling 800-772-1213.

Going through the application process, which involves many people and many forms, can take several months. Take a few deep breaths to stay calm, especially if you're waiting on the telephone or in line. Here's where your organization of your medical records will pay off. (And now you know why I harp throughout this book about the need to keep a hep C notebook, which I explain in Chapter 5.) See the sidebar "Getting a head start on the disability application" so you can gather the information you need for your application. Good luck!

Saving for Yourself and Your Family

The knowledge that you have a long-term illness can make you think about the financial future for yourself and your loved ones. Planning ahead is smart, and especially so when you have hepatitis C. If you can, do it while you're still working and feeling well. Later, you may be on treatment or have more severe hepatitis C, and you'll be mighty glad that your finances are in order.

Getting life insurance

Life insurance is a set of payments you make now to provide a fund for your family after you die. You may be offered life insurance through your job, or you may wish to purchase a policy on your own.

How much, if any, trouble you have getting a new life insurance policy depends on the features of your hepatitis C illness and the insurance company you're dealing with. Most life insurance companies look at your health to determine eligibility. Insurers want to know whether your disease is under control or whether your health is declining. Tell them if you've been successful with interferon treatment or if you have only mild symptoms that haven't gotten worse.

If you do have cirrhosis, liver failure, or liver cancer, life insurance companies are unlikely to offer you a traditional policy. Here's what you can do:

- ✔ Look around at different companies; policies may differ.

- ✔ Consider saving money in other ways.

- ✔ Investigate insurance policies through your employer or associations that are "guaranteed" and that don't ask health questions.

Planning for the inevitable

Getting old and dying are inevitable, with or without hepatitis C. With hepatitis C, what you don't know is how your hepatitis C will affect your ability to work and whether it will develop into a serious illness and premature death. You'll feel better if you know that you have taken care of the loose ends of your estate and finances, so consider this advice:

- ✔ Make sure you'll have the savings you might need later on, when you may not be able to work.

- ✔ Make sure that you've done all you can to provide for your children and their educational needs.

Take a look at *Estate Planning For Dummies,* by N. Brian Caverly and Jordan S. Simon (Wiley), for info on net worth, wills, trust funds, and more. Also consult a qualified financial planner or lawyer for advice on your personal situation.

Part IV

Considering Different Groups with Hepatitis C

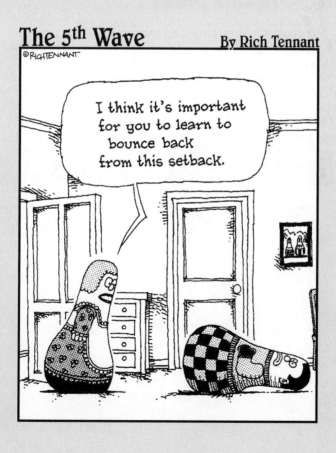

The 5th Wave   By Rich Tennant

©RICHTENNANT

I think it's important for you to learn to bounce back from this setback.

In this part . . .

Hepatitis C virus knows no barriers: It infects people of both genders and all ages, nationalities, and races. This part covers specific recommendations or problems that exist for different groups with hep C, including children, African Americans, and Latinos. I also discuss issues specific to men and to women, who have special concerns if they wish to have children while infected. In addition, this part has information for veterans who may have been infected during active duty. And if you're a friend or family member of a person living with hepatitis C, you can find information that will enable you to best help your loved one.

Chapter 17

Helping Kids with Hepatitis C

● ●

In This Chapter

▶ Knowing the risk factors and symptoms of hep C in children

▶ Considering the possibility of mother-to-child transmission

▶ Getting your child tested

▶ Specifying ways to treat your child

▶ Enjoying childhood despite hepatitis C

● ●

*I*f you're a parent, finding out that your child has a chronic illness like hepatitis C can seem overwhelming. The good news is that children generally have a milder hepatitis C disease and are more likely to eradicate the virus on their own. But some children do have symptoms, and as they age, they have a chance of developing inflammation, scarring, and even cirrhosis or liver cancer. Getting good medical care is important so that you stay on top of your child's health and find out about the latest medical treatments.

Mothers with the hepatitis C virus pass the infection to their baby in about 5 percent of births, and having two people in the family with the disease can be doubly hard. However, eating well (Chapter 11), avoiding toxins (Chapter 12), and reducing stress (Chapter 13) are important ways that help both children and adults with hepatitis C continue to enjoy a healthy life.

In this chapter, I describe what's known about hepatitis C in children and give you information and suggestions so you can help your child and your family.

Looking at Hep C in Children

Experts estimate that between 100,000 and 150,000 children in the United States are currently infected with hepatitis C virus. Around the world, approximately 10,000 cases of mother-to-child transmission occur each year.

Children respond somewhat differently to hepatitis C infection than adults, and some differences depend on the child's age. In most cases, disease progression is milder in children: More children get rid of the virus on their own without medication, and children are less likely to have symptoms and problems.

Unfortunately, chronic hepatitis C can cause disease at any time, and the chances of this happening increase as your child ages. By carefully monitoring your children, your doctor can spot the disease when it comes out of hiding and starts to cause damage. At that time, your doctor may recommend starting antiviral treatment to halt the disease progression (see the "Deciding on Treatment" section, later in the chapter).

Overall, the disease progression in children is similar to that in adults: liver inflammation followed by fibrosis (scarring), which if unstopped could become cirrhosis. Liver cancer is also possible in children.

Infants, who are defined as children less than 1 year, can develop cirrhosis and need a liver transplant to survive, but that happens only rarely.

So the prognosis for children with hepatitis C is generally better than that for adults. Some treatments are approved for use in children (see the section "Deciding on Treatment," later in this chapter), and medical studies are looking at the long-term safety and effectiveness of hepatitis C treatment for children. Treatments available in the future should be even more promising for children.

Defining risk factors in children

Children have the same risk factors for hep C virus transmission as adults, with the additional possibility of acquiring the hep C virus during birth. Here are the ways a child might get the hepatitis C virus:

- ✓ **Transmission from mother to child:** This is now the most likely cause of hepatitis C infection in children. See the section "Transmitting Hepatitis C from Mother to Child," later in the chapter.

- ✓ **Exposure to blood transfusion or organ transplant before 1992:** Because the blood supply is now tested for hep C, the chances of getting infected from a transfusion are 1 per 1 million units of blood. If your child had a transfusion before 1992, there is a chance that he or she got hep C from that exposure. Organs are also now tested for hepatitis C.

✔ **Transfusion of clotting factors before 1987:** If a child with hemophilia or another clotting factor deficiency received clotting factor (from pooled blood) with hepatitis C virus before 1987, he may have gotten the hepatitis C virus. Clotting factors are now protected against hepatitis C virus and other viruses, like HIV and hepatitis B.

✔ **Member of a household with hepatitis C:** This is probably the least likely route of exposure for a child to get hepatitis C, but this method of transmission is theoretically possible if a child used a razor or toothbrush that had infected blood.

Inform your pediatrician if your child has any risk factors for hepatitis C. Testing children or adolescents who have risk factors allows earlier treatment and management of hepatitis C.

For older children, the paths to hepatitis C transmission can resemble those of adults even more closely. Check out all the transmission info in Chapter 2, but keep these means in mind for older children:

✔ Injection drug use

✔ Sexual activity with exposure to blood

✔ Sharing of paper currency or straws for intranasal cocaine use

✔ Tattoos or piercings in unsanitary situations

Examining symptoms in children

Symptoms in children are similar to those in adults, but the tricky part is that younger children are less able to define their symptoms, and they may have fewer symptoms. Watch for the following:

✔ Flu-like symptoms (achiness, fever, diarrhea, or nausea)

✔ Tiredness

✔ Loss of appetite or weight loss

✔ Dark-colored urine

✔ Light-colored feces

✔ Stomach pain, especially in the upper-right abdominal area

✔ Jaundice (yellowing of the eyes and skin)

Infants under 1 also may have an enlarged liver or spleen, grow more slowly, or fail to gain weight.

Children may have no symptoms, but hep C can eventually lead to a life-threatening illness, including cirrhosis, liver failure, or liver cancer. If your child has any of the symptoms of hepatitis C — or any of the risk factors outlined earlier — contact your pediatrician. Remember that earlier testing leads to earlier treatment and more effective disease management.

Transmitting Hepatitis C from Mother to Child

About 5 out of every 100 babies (5 percent) born to a mother with hep C RNA (see Chapter 6) in her blood will get the virus. Because this number is relatively small, women with hepatitis C aren't specifically counseled to avoid pregnancy. Whether or not to become pregnant is an individual decision for each couple to make.

Here's some information culled from research studies about mother-to-child transmission of hep C:

- ✔ A factor that's related to transmission of hep C to your children is your viral load. If you have more virus in your blood, as measured by hep C RNA tests (see Chapter 6), you're more likely to transmit the virus.

- ✔ Infection with hepatitis C virus happens at the time of birth. To reduce the chance of being exposed to the mother's blood at birth, some experts recommend an elective Caesarean section. Either a vaginal birth or emergency Caesarean section can bring the baby in contact with the mother's blood. Researchers are looking at the pros and cons of this choice. Discuss your options for birth with your partner, gynecologist, and liver specialist.

- ✔ Other procedures during pregnancy or birth that might expose the baby to mom's blood should be avoided or practiced with caution:

  - • **Amniocentesis:** This test uses a needle to access the *amniotic fluid* (the clear fluid that surrounds the fetus) during pregnancy to look for birth defects.

  - • **Fetal scalp monitoring:** This method of checking on the baby's heart rate with scalp electrodes could put tiny cuts in the infant's head through which hep C virus could pass.

- ✔ The hepatitis C virus has been found in breast milk, but there's no evidence for transmission through breastfeeding. Medical experts recommend that women with hepatitis C breastfeed their babies because of the benefits of breastfeeding for the child. If you have cracked or bleeding nipples, however, you should refrain from breastfeeding.

✔ If you have co-infection with human immunodeficiency virus (HIV), studies show that your chance of passing your hep C to your children is 17 percent (versus 5 percent with hepatitis C alone).

Testing Children

Needles, blood work, and biopsies are particularly difficult for children and families. Infants, toddlers, and even older children won't initially understand why they have to be subjected to such scary and uncomfortable events. But kids can get used to the procedures — and you can take steps to help increase their comfort level.

You may want to plan some treat for your child before or after the testing. For example, you could make a special meal for your child (but go easy on the junk food, which isn't so good for the liver!). Even better, let your kid get involved with the pre- and post-procedure planning:

✔ **Let your infant/toddler hold a special stuffed animal, doll, or blanket:** This connection to a familiar object gives the child some comfort and feeling of control during the injection process.

✔ **Let your child pick out something special to wear:** A special shirt, ribbon, bracelet, and so on may help. Maybe your child simply wants to wear a special color that she feels good about.

✔ **Let your child pick a special CD or videotape:** Listening to a favorite singer or watching a favorite movie may help take the child's mind off the procedure.

Check out the section "Explaining hepatitis C to children," later in the chapter, for more tips on helping kids through the testing process. But you also need to feel comfortable to help ease the anxiety in the family when you're facing tests and procedures. And the first step to being more comfortable is getting the facts.

Hep C virus tests

The two basic blood tests for hep C virus look for antibody or RNA. I cover general information about hep C virus tests in Chapter 6, but the following section explains the specifics related to kids.

Anti-hepatitis C antibody

If your child is older than 18 months old, the anti-hepatitis C antibody test is an accurate way to test for exposure to the hepatitis C virus. But your baby's positive anti-hepatitis C antibody test can be a false positive if the test is performed before your child is 18 months old. The reason is that mothers pass their own antibodies on to their children, where they can linger for up to 18 months. If the mother has hepatitis C antibodies, these are present in her young children. This is nature's way of protecting children until they produce their own antibodies.

Unfortunately, the antibodies that are detected by the anti-hepatitis C test aren't the ones that protect against infection.

Even if the mother or child's virus has all but disappeared, due to treatment or luck, antibodies may still be present in the blood. Antibodies against hepatitis C are still produced after the virus infection has been eradicated.

To see whether you still have the virus, you need to have an RNA test.

Hep C RNA tests

An RNA test is used to look for the presence of the hepatitis C virus. Both types of RNA test, qualitative or quantitative, look to see whether your child has an active hepatitis C infection. Your child will be tested for hep C RNA as follows:

- ✔ **Infants** born to mothers positive for hepatitis C can be tested at 2 months and then again at 5 or 6 months. (Antibody tests aren't reliable at this early age due to the presence of maternal antibodies.)

- ✔ **Toddlers and older children** are tested for hep C RNA if their antibody tests are positive.

Yearly, or more often if your child has symptoms, your pediatrician will repeat an RNA test, along with liver enzyme/function tests, as described in the next section. This regular testing enables the doctor to keep on top of your child's illness. The RNA test tells the doctor if your kid has eradicated his virus.

At some point, your child may have the anti-hepatitis C antibody, but the RNA test shows no virus. This result means that your child has naturally eradicated his hepatitis C infection!

Your kid's doctor may perform viral load tests (quantitative RNA tests) to determine the amount of virus your child has. Note though that viral load doesn't always correlate with how serious the disease will be; it's a measure of how much virus your child has.

Liver tests in children

The alanine aminotransferase (ALT) and aspartate aminotransferase (AST) liver enzyme tests (discussed in Chapter 7) are recommended for children, although the normal levels aren't as clearly defined as for adults, and results may vary at times.

Children who have any liver damage (indicated by elevated levels of ALT or AST) need to see a pediatric gastroenterologist or hepatologist, who is experienced in treating liver disorders. (See Chapter 5 for more about finding and communicating with a doctor.)

If your child has elevated ALT levels, your doctor may want to perform a biopsy. If your child needs a liver biopsy, try to explain the procedure in simple terms — if your child is old enough. Here are some things your child can expect:

- ✔ No eating or drinking after midnight the night before the biopsy
- ✔ Getting blood drawn on the morning of the biopsy
- ✔ Being sedated for the procedure (see Chapter 7 for a description of the liver biopsy procedure in adults)
- ✔ Getting checked after the biopsy to make sure everything is okay

Also let your child know that he can eat after he wakes up and that he may have to stay overnight in the hospital.

In addition to liver enzyme tests and biopsies, your doctor may also perform these tests, covered in Chapter 7:

- ✔ **Alpha-fetoprotein test:** Some doctors use this test to monitor the progression of liver disease in children.
- ✔ **Ultrasound test:** Your doctor may also perform this test to obtain a baseline to use if your child ever develops liver disease down the road.

Deciding on Treatment

Decisions to treat children aren't as clear-cut as they are for adults. For one thing, most medications haven't been tested in children, so their safety and effectiveness isn't well established. Another factor is that the course of hepatitis C disease in children is slower and milder, so the impetus to treat earlier rather than later isn't as great for children as it is for adults. Some doctors don't treat children until they turn 18. Other doctors treat at an earlier age, but this is usually decided on a case-by-case basis. For young people with hepatitis C, there's room for optimism, because new products with potentially greater safety and effectiveness are in the development pipeline.

The only treatment currently approved by the FDA for use in children is Schering-Plough's Intron A (interferon alpha-2b), which I discuss in Chapter 8, and ribavirin (Rebetol). Intron A, like the other interferons, is administered through injection. Intron A isn't a pegylated form of interferon and must be injected more often (three times a week). Ribavirin is taken by adults in pill form, and a bubble-gum-flavored liquid ribavirin (Rebetol) is now available for children.

Giving a child an injection, or going to get a blood draw can be challenging! Parents of Kids with Infectious Diseases (PKIDs) offers tips on its Web site (www.pkids.org) to help you and your child deal with the injection process. Here are a few of those suggestions:

✔ Speak to your doctor about using EMLA Cream to reduce pain at the injection site.

✔ Keep your child away from the injection materials and injection room until time for the injection, so he's not worrying about the upcoming shot all day.

✔ Pick a sanitary and quiet place in the home to do injections. The kitchen and bathroom probably aren't the best places.

You can also try to distract your kid by talking about something else, letting her watch TV, or asking her to wiggle her toes.

If you want to treat your child with complementary or alternative medicine (CAM), find a healthcare practitioner who's knowledgeable about liver disease and children. And tell your pediatrician or pediatric gastroenterologist about any herbs or other treatments that your child is taking.

Don't be tempted to treat your child yourself with any product, especially one that is intended for adults. Children react differently and to lower doses of herbs than adults.

Experiencing Childhood with Hepatitis C

 From a medical standpoint, hepatitis C shouldn't affect your child's ability to participate in usual childhood activities, including sports activities.

Explaining hepatitis C to children

You're likely reading this book right now to find out more about hepatitis C and, therefore, to become more comfortable and confident in dealing with the illness. Children (especially older children) can also benefit from information. Talk with your doctors and nurses about how you and they can best explain the disease and procedures to children.

Here are some typical questions your child might ask, along with simplified ways of explaining hep C and testing procedures to young children. Modify them for your own use.

✔ **What is a liver?**

 Inside the body, here under your right rib, is a liver. (You can poke gently in the general area of your child's body to explain where it is. You also may want to go to the supermarket and show your child a beef or chicken liver.) *Your liver helps you digest food and get rid of bad chemicals.*

✔ **What is a virus?**

 A virus is a tiny infection (germ) that can make you sick.

✔ **What is the hepatitis C virus?**

 The hepatitis C virus is a tiny germ that infects your liver.

✔ **What is hepatitis C disease?**

 When the hepatitis C virus stays in your body, you can get sick. Your liver may not work so well.

✔ **What is a blood test?**

 The doctor needs to see a little bit of your blood to see if you have the virus or are getting sick.

✔ **Why do you use needles?**

 The needle goes into your vein (very quickly) to get a little blood.

✔ **What is a liver biopsy?**

The doctor is going to take a really small piece of your liver to look at under the microscope. She can look at your liver and then give you medicine if you need it to get better.

Protecting the household

Household infection is uncommon, but you still need to take precautions to avoid exposing others to any danger. But don't become overly paranoid, because this type of fear can spread to your child and others. Protection from hep C in the household is just a matter of common sense: Avoid exposure to blood. Because blood is normally inside our bodies, protecting yourself is relatively easy.

When someone in your household has hepatitis C, whether it is only one child or a parent and a child, teach your family not to share household items, including the following:

✔ Shaving razors

✔ Manicure items (such as nail clippers or cuticle scissors)

✔ Toothbrushes and toothpaste

Encourage everyone in your household to separate their personal items from other people's things by using small bags or plastic boxes with children's names or buying different colors or brands of items to make it easy to keep them apart. If all family members keep their toothpaste and toothbrushes separate from the others, then the children or adults with hepatitis C don't feel singled out.

When your child is old enough, he'll be able to understand that he must keep his cuts covered up. Try to keep bandages nearby to cover any cuts or wounds. Any objects soiled with blood should be carefully disposed of and not left around to infect others. Try to give your kids this advice in a way that emphasizes hygiene for the whole family, and not with shame or paranoia. Here are some other tips on keeping things safe at home:

✔ If you have children sleeping over, have extra toothbrushing supplies on hand so that no one needs to share.

✔ Teach your children about razors and safe disposal of sanitary items *before* puberty sets in and your children have already started shaving or menstruating.

✔ Just as your child must be aware of the need to keep his cuts covered up, other children in the household also need to know of this potential risk so they don't inadvertently expose themselves to blood.

✔ Use latex gloves to clean up any wounds or accidents involving blood from a person with hep C. Some people use this precaution with any exposure to blood.

Telling other people your child has hep C

The question of whom to tell about your child's hep C and how to do it isn't easy. Talk to your spouse, and plan in advance whom you want to tell and when and how you want to tell them.

You don't have to tell anyone about your child's hep C, but you'll probably want to notify healthcare workers so your child can get the appropriate medical care. You may feel ethically obligated to tell other people who might be exposed to your child's blood when he gets the usual childhood scrapes and cuts from normal playing and roughhousing. If you're concerned about whom to tell and what the ramifications might be for your child, speak with a lawyer.

All schools, childcare centers, camps, and other institutions are required by law to practice universal precautions when dealing with any person's blood or body fluids. (Universal precautions involve wearing latex gloves, and goggles if necessary, to protect the skin when dealing with blood or body fluids.) These safety precautions protect others from getting a bloodborne virus, such as hepatitis C or even HIV. Because some children can be virus carriers without even knowing it, *every* child's blood or body fluid should be treated as though it might be infected.

A common concern is that some individuals— perhaps babysitters, mothers of other children, or even other children — may not know or practice safe techniques when dealing with your child's blood. You can decide on a case-by-case basis whom to tell after evaluating their potential risk of infection. You can also ask people to keep the information confidential. Here are some tips for telling people about your kid's hep C:

✔ Prepare yourself by having a script of what you'll say, and have answers to possible questions.

✔ Speak to your spouse so that both of you are prepared and can support each other.

✔ Have some information leaflets about hep C to give to people (see the resources listed in Chapter 22).

✔ Inform folks that hep C isn't easily spread; it only spreads through blood. Everyone should take precautions if exposed to his blood (just as they would if exposed to anyone's blood): Use latex gloves to dress any wounds, dispose of blood-soaked items with care, and cover all your child's cuts.

✔ Remind them that your child deserves to be treated with as much love and respect as any child.

When you tell people about your child's hep C, you face the risk of discrimination. I hope that you don't encounter this problem, which usually results from ignorance and fear, but discrimination does sometimes occur. Discrimination or stigma is one of the most painful things that a child with hepatitis C may go through.

To avoid this potential problem, some parents may opt not to tell anyone about their child's hepatitis C. Other parents seek legal advice and inform certain select individuals: babysitters, school nurses, and so on. For more advice, speak to your doctor, find a support group of parents of children with hepatitis C (or other infectious diseases), and check out Chapter 15 for related information on stigma.

To get support and information on issues including discrimination, check out a great organization called Parents of Kids with Infectious Diseases (phone toll-free, 877-557-5437, or visit the Web site at www. pkids.org); it has a listserv for parents of kids with infectious diseases. If you can't find a support group near your home, you can communicate with other parents by e-mail or telephone, or start your own group!

Tell people that hepatitis C isn't easily spread and that common activities, such as changing diapers, hugging, sharing food or water, swimming in the same pool, or even sneezing, won't spread the virus. Some people confuse hepatitis C and hepatitis A (which is spread through diapers, food, and water). Educate yourself on the differences among the different hepatitis C viruses (which I describe in Chapter 2) so you can inform others.

Using artistic expression

You may want to try letting your child explain to you through art how he feels about the having hepatitis or liver disease. Because many children (and adults) love artwork, ask your child to draw a liver or what it feels like to have hepatitis disease, having tests, and so on. Give him paper, crayons, paint, pencils, and any other art supplies that may help him express himself. Don't judge the artwork, and always ask whether he wants to display it somewhere in your home.

Keeping your child healthy

Children with hep C are advised to avoid toxins, eat healthy foods, refrain from alcohol and drugs, and get vaccinated against hepatitis A and B. Here are some specific tips for ways parents can help their kids stay healthy:

- ✔ **Protect them from toxins.** Because a child may live with chronic hepatitis C infection for many decades, avoiding toxic exposures that can also damage the liver becomes especially important. (See Chapter 12 for a discussion of dangerous substances.) As children get older, talk to them about the dangers of smoking, drinking, and using drugs, particularly if they have hepatitis C.

- ✔ **Serve healthy foods and encourage drinking plenty of water.** Your doctor may have recommendations for your infant or child about foods that are easier to digest, especially if the youngster is having digestive troubles. (See Chapter 11 for the scoop about good nutrition.) The most important advice may be to avoid certain trouble foods, such as fatty and sugary foods. Introduce your children at a young age to fresh fruits and vegetables. Give them whole grains and organic foods, if you can.

- ✔ **Get your child vaccinated against hepatitis A and B.** Hepatitis A and B can spread easily in childcare settings. Talk to your pediatrician about getting your child immunized against both of these viruses, which also damage the liver. If your baby has hep C, being co-infected with another type of hepatitis virus can be dangerous. See Chapter 2 for more on the problems of co-infection.

Dealing with emotional issues

Having a child with hep C can be a huge strain on the parents and siblings of a child who is ill. You may be filled with worry about your child's future or overwhelmed by dealing with your own issues if you yourself have hepatitis C. Get help and advice from your doctor or support group, or contact Parents of Kids with Infectious Diseases (PKIDs). You also may want to consider getting professional help for yourself and your family.

Letting your child have a happy childhood experience can be a help for children and parents! PKIDs has a summer-camp program for kids with hepatitis B or C. At two different camps, one in upstate New York and one in Florida, children from ages 8 to 16 with chronic hepatitis C can experience fun and meet other children with the disease, all while having expert medical attention. Contact www.pkids.org or call 877-557-5437 for more information.

Chapter 18

Special Groups with Hepatitis C

. . . .

In This Chapter

▶ Considering gender differences

▶ Looking at the African American and Latino populations

▶ Understanding issues involving veterans and healthcare workers

▶ Assessing the needs of those with HIV, drug users, and prisoners

. . . .

*I*n this chapter, I've gathered information for certain groups to make it easier to find. Use this information to help yourself or a loved one. Because this chapter (or this book) doesn't have enough room to give individualized information for every possible person with hep C, I focus on covering info that applies specifically to men, women, and the two largest minority groups with hep C in the United States: African Americans and Latinos. (See Chapter 17 for special information on pregnancy and children with hepatitis C.)

I also provide information here for groups that are traditionally shunned by society: people who are or have been in jail, have injected illegal drugs, or have human immunodeficiency virus (HIV). The reality is that hepatitis C infection is very high in these groups where information and resources to deal with the physical, emotional, and financial impact of the disease are often in short supply.

Gender and Hepatitis C

Whether you are male or female, hepatitis C can be devastating in its effects on your health and your life. Each gender has some specific problems that are related to effects of hep C on hormones.

The liver helps process the female and male sex hormones, estrogen and testosterone, respectively. So it's no surprise to find that when the liver is damaged by hepatitis C, your hormone levels can get out of whack. Hormones play a role in your sexual desire and your ability to perform sexually (see Chapter 15 for more on this issue). They also function in reproduction and a woman's menstrual cycle. The actual effects of hepatitis C on your hormones depend on how well your liver is functioning. If you have cirrhosis, and your liver function is impaired, then the problems with hormones can be more serious.

Birth control

In considering birth control methods, ask yourself the following questions:

- ✔ Will it protect you or your partner from pregnancy and/or sexually transmitted diseases?
- ✔ Will it protect your sex partner from your hep C?
- ✔ Is the method of birth control safe for you and your partner?

The latex condom, for example, can protect against sexually transmitted diseases like hepatitis C and human immunodeficiency virus, but it's not as effective in preventing pregnancy as the birth control pill (which doesn't protect against sexually transmitted diseases and may have health risks for women with hep C).

During hepatitis C drug treatment, you must use two reliable methods of birth control to avoid problems of birth defects associated with the drugs.

For women

Hepatitis C infection and liver disease can affect women's hormones, premenopausal and postmenopausal symptoms, and perhaps even fertility. More studies are needed to fully understand and treat women's issues and to understand how women's hormones may affect the progression of liver disease.

Premenstrual syndrome and menstruation

Hep C can cause changes in your periods or premenstrual symptoms (PMS), but it may be difficult to sort out whether the symptoms are a result of hep C or PMS. Moodiness, achiness, depression, and fatigue can go along with premenstrual syndrome, hepatitis C, or even menopause.

During menstruation, when you're actively bleeding, anyone exposed to your blood can become infected if you have the hep C virus in your blood at this time (as determined by tests described in Chapter 6). During menstruation, protect your loved ones by:

✔ Practicing safer sex (by using a latex condom) or abstaining from sex. Talk to your sex partner about your hep C so he can protect himself (see Chapter 15).

✔ Safely disposing of your sanitary products by wrapping them properly so that no one in your household will inadvertently be exposed to your blood.

In the later stages of hepatitis C, your body may not tolerate the hormones (estrogen and progesterone) in birth control pills, so discuss birth control options with your doctor. Some doctors recommend a progesterone-only pill.

Pregnancy and childbirth

You can still have children and breastfeed when you have hep C, although there's a small (about 5 percent) risk of passing the hep C virus to your child during birth. As I discuss in Chapter 17, the decision to have children when you have hep C is intensely personal. Discuss this topic with your partner and healthcare professional. Although hep C is present in breast milk, the virus isn't thought to spread this way. You're advised to refrain from breastfeeding, however, if your nipples are cracked or bleeding.

Menopause

Your estrogen levels change after menopause, and many women experience problems like night sweats, foggy thinking, moodiness, fatigue, and osteoporosis (thinning bones) that can also be symptoms of hep C or cirrhosis.

Some women go on hormone replacement therapy to help with symptoms of menopause, but this must be done with care if you have hep C. Your doctor can help you make the best decision after weighing the pros and cons of this treatment. Chapters 11 and 13 have advice that also may help ease some of the symptoms.

Your doctor should monitor you for osteoporosis, because both menopause and cirrhosis can contribute to this problem.

For men

Men also experience hormonal difficulties, especially in the later stages of liver disease. Decreased levels of testosterone can lead to the following:

> ✔ Enlarged breasts (*gynecomastia*)
>
> ✔ Sexual difficulties, including lack of interest in sex, problems with erection (erectile dysfunction), and ejaculation problems

Problems with your sexual functioning can affect your relationships and self-esteem. See your physician for medical advice. I discuss loss of interest in sex in more depth in Chapter 15.

In the United States, more men than women have hepatitis C. Some of the risk factors leading to the infection — using street drugs, spending time in jail, and serving in Vietnam — are believed to account for this difference. Men are also more likely to develop serious liver disease than women. Different theories try to explain why men are more likely to get cirrhosis, including the following:

> ✔ Men drink more alcohol, which damages the liver, than women.
>
> ✔ The female hormone estrogen may protect women to some extent from developing liver disease.

Ethnicity and Hepatitis C

If you're a non-Caucasian person with hepatitis C, you may want to ask your prospective liver doctor a question in addition to those listed in Chapter 5: Have you treated women or men of my ethnic group with hepatitis C?

Depending on your ethnicity, you may have a different way of responding to the interferon treatment. Because interferon treatment has serious side effects, you must evaluate the risks of the treatment in light of its potential benefit to you. Also, as new studies become available, recommendations for treating specific groups of people are being made.

African Americans

Researchers are paying increased attention to hep C in African Americans. Here's what's known at this point:

> ✔ An estimated 10 percent of African American males between the ages of 40 and 49 have the hep C virus.
>
> ✔ Overall, 3.2 percent of African Americans are estimated to have hep C (compared with 1.5 percent of whites and 2.1 percent of Latinos).

✔ African Americans have a higher rate of genotype 1 infection, which is more resistant to treatment (see Chapter 8).

✔ African Americans have a lower responsiveness to interferon treatment than non-African Americans.

✔ Disease progression may be slower in African Americans than in Caucasians. African Americans have lower levels of the ALT (alanine aminotransferase) enzyme, which is used to measure liver damage, and less fibrosis (liver scarring) than non-African Americans. (For more on ALT, see Chapter 7.)

✔ African American men are more likely to develop liver cancer.

 As more African Americans are included in clinical trials, researchers are identifying the best types of treatment options. Make sure that your doctor is up-to-date on the studies involving African Americans and recommendations for treatment. Chapter 8 covers treatment issues in general.

Latinos and Hispanics

About 2.1 percent (or 1 out of 50) of Hispanics are infected with hepatitis C virus. The U.S. Centers for Disease Control and Prevention (CDC) defines a Hispanic or Latino as a person who may be *any* race and is of Cuban, Mexican, Puerto Rican, South or Central American, or other Spanish culture or origin. Hispanics of all races make up about 12.5 percent of the U.S. population.

Studies on the effectiveness of interferon drug treatments for Hispanics are even fewer than those for African Americans. Researchers believe that the effectiveness of combination interferon treatment in Hispanics is dependent on the hep C genotype.

 Language can be a barrier to getting information out about hep C and its prevention in the Latino communities. The CDC, American Liver Foundation, and other organizations provide information in Spanish (see Chapter 22 for resources). Another source of information is LOLA (Latino Organization for Liver Awareness). Contact the group through its Web site, www.lola-national.org, or call 888-367-5652.

Veterans

Veterans in the United States are more likely to be infected with hepatitis C than nonveterans. The U.S. Veterans Administration (VA) reports that around 5.4 percent of veterans in the VA healthcare system are positive for the hep C virus. The VA says that veterans are more at risk of having hep C if they've injected illegal drugs, served in the Vietnam War, been in jail for more than 48 hours, or received a tattoo. The VA has set up a Web site at `http://hepatitis.va.gov` specifically for vets with hep C.

Ways that veterans could have been exposed to hepatitis C include

- Blood or body fluid exposure by healthcare or combat personnel
- Contamination of vaccinations or immune globulin (which are antibodies from pooled blood that is given to boost your immunity to certain infections)
- Sharing shaving razors or other nonsterile instruments

A point of controversy is whether multidose vaccinations (in which a jet gun was used to perform multiple vaccinations on many different people) served as a source of infection with hepatitis C during the Vietnam War.

Healthcare Workers

If you're a healthcare, emergency medical, or public safety worker, the CDC recommends testing for hepatitis C infection after exposure to HCV-positive blood through a puncture of your skin by a needlestick or other sharp object.

If you're exposed to a needlestick or sharps, and the contaminating blood is infected with hep C, you have about a 2 percent chance of getting infected. Exposure is also possible if infected blood comes in contact with your mucosal membranes (mouth, eyes, and nose), although infection by this route is unlikely.

See a hepatitis specialist for specific treatment guidelines if you're exposed to hepatitis C on the job. Some doctors may consider early treatment, which at the time of this writing is not FDA-approved, but early studies indicate that treatment is more likely to eradicate the virus at this early stage of infection.

People Co-Infected with HIV and Hepatitis C

Because HIV is spread through blood and body fluids, and hepatitis C is spread through blood, many folks have both viruses. Here are some other facts on the transmission of these viruses:

✔ HIV can spread through sex, and any type of sex that involves exposure to blood can also spread the hepatitis C virus (see Chapter 2).

✔ Injection of street drugs is a major route of both HIV and hepatitis C infection, and leads to most cases of co-infection.

✔ Hemophiliacs and others who received infected blood or blood products may also have been exposed to both viruses.

✔ HIV spreads more easily from mother to child than the hepatitis C virus, and HIV can also be transmitted through breastfeeding.

Hepatitis B can also be spread in the same way as HIV, and a person can be co-infected with both hepatitis B and hepatitis C (see Chapter 2) or hepatitis B and HIV.

Having two viruses makes it more challenging for your body and your medical team to fight each infection. HIV causes an immunodeficiency disease, acquired immunodeficiency syndrome (AIDS). When you have AIDS, your body is less able to fight the hepatitis C virus. Another complication is that the drugs used to fight HIV infection can be harmful to your liver, which may already be damaged from the hepatitis C virus. Your doctor will monitor your liver for any additional damage and make changes in your HIV medication if necessary.

Treatment strategies for people with HIV who are co-infected with hepatitis C virus have improved as studies look at this special population. Peginterferon plus ribavirin is the current treatment of choice if you're co-infected with HIV and hepatitis C.

For current information on HIV, hepatitis C, and co-infection studies, check out the Web sites of HIVandHepatitis.com (www.hiv andhepatitis.com) and the National AIDS Treatment Advocacy Project (www.natap.org). You can also contact NATAP toll-free at 888-266-2827.

People Who Inject Illegal Drugs

Sharing needles or other drug paraphernalia remains the likeliest form of transmission. Taking drugs through your nose can also spread hepatitis C if you share paraphernalia for snorting. Many people who use illegal drugs are outside the conventional healthcare system and may not receive adequate treatment. See Chapter 16 for suggestions on getting healthcare if you're not insured.

Agencies that deal with *harm reduction* accept that drug use is part of the world and work to reduce the harm that comes from illicit drug use, including hepatitis C infection. Rather than punish or judge drug users, harm reduction aims to empower drug users to help themselves without minimizing the problems that drug use causes. For more about this topic, visit the Web site www.harmreduction.org. And I discuss the problems of drug use and hepatitis C infection in Chapter 12.

People in Prison

Millions of Americans are currently housed in correctional facilities. Experts estimate that an average of 30 to 35 percent of all people in prison have hepatitis C. Many people in jail have injected illegal drugs or engaged in commercial sex (prostitution), which are two routes of hepatitis C infection. If you get a tattoo or piercing while in a correctional facility, you also can get infected with the hepatitis C virus.

Whether or not you'll be offered testing and treatment while in prison depends on each individual facility. If you have hepatitis C and fulfill the criteria for treatment at that facility (see Chapter 8 for information on drug treatment), the doctor will want to make sure that you'll be able to complete the drug regimen, which may be a year or more. That means that you may have to forgo early parole or release from prison so that you can complete the medical treatment before leaving the facility.

If you don't finish treatment, the problem is that you might not have health insurance to continue treatment as soon as you leave prison, and completing the entire course of treatment is especially important with hep C medications.

Many prisoners also have HIV or mental illness alongside their hep C. If you have these conditions, you need proper treatment for these illnesses before or during your treatment for hepatitis C virus.

Some prisons offer information on hep C risk reduction through education about avoiding drug use and practicing safer injection drug use and safer sex. For more information about hepatitis C in prisons, check out the Web site for the National Hepatitis C Prison Coalition, www.hcvinprison.org.

Chapter 19

For Family and Friends

- -

In This Chapter

▶ Finding out all you can about hepatitis C

▶ Keeping yourself healthy

▶ Serving on the support team

▶ Sharing a household

▶ Considering sexual partners

▶ Finding creative ways to help out

- -

*T*he hepatitis C virus can infect anyone: your husband, best friend, or co-worker. When you find out about your loved one's illness, you may feel confused and scared. He or she may be in the early stages of illness or have advanced liver disease and be unable to work. What will happen to the person? How can you help?

Whether you're the primary caretaker or a long-distance relative, your support can help. In this chapter, I give you the lowdown on how to educate yourself about hep C, how to help the person you care about, and how to keep yourself well too.

Enlightening Yourself about Hepatitis C

The more you know about hepatitis C, the more you can help your friend, partner, or family member deal with this long-term chronic illness. Get reliable information from different sources. This book has chapters on just about all aspects of living with hepatitis C. Consult the resources I provide within individual chapters and in Chapter 22 for additional information.

Here are some topics that you may want to know more about:

✔ The ways that hepatitis C is and isn't transmitted (see Chapter 2)

✔ The different types of diseases associated with hepatitis C (see Chapter 4)

✔ Different treatment options (see Chapters 8, 9, and 10)

✔ Maintaining a healthy lifestyle (see Chapters 11 and 13 for more about nutrition and exercise, respectively)

Consider volunteering for your local branch of the American Liver Foundation or another hepatitis C–related organization. These organizations can always use volunteers for a variety of tasks. See Chapter 22 for some contact info for these groups.

Taking Care of Yourself

Who takes care of the caretakers? If you give too much to other people and don't take care of yourself, you could suffer from early burnout and then be unavailable when you're really needed. Just as airlines tell passengers to give themselves oxygen in an emergency before giving oxygen masks to children, your first priority is taking care of yourself.

Rather than put this section last, I put it early in this chapter so that you remember to keep all of your own support in place while helping your loved one with hepatitis C. Ask yourself these questions to help ensure that you take care of yourself:

✔ Are you taking care of your own physical needs? Do you get enough sleep, eat well, and exercise regularly?

✔ Do you have someone to talk to? You might feel worried or frustrated about your friend and need a supportive friend or professional therapist to help you.

✔ Do you have time off from being the caregiver? Sometimes you won't be able to help as much as you would like. Figure out how to use the word *no* when you need to.

If you stay in good emotional, mental, and physical shape, your loved one will benefit much more from your calm and healthy attitude.

If you're the primary caretaker, assemble a team of helpers so all the responsibilities don't fall on your shoulders.

Being Part of a Support Team

Everyone with hepatitis C needs a support team. The support team for people with hepatitis C includes family and friends, healthcare providers, and other professionals, such as financial advisers and social workers. Although one person may "lead" the team, a *group* of people should be providing support. For example, some family and friends may be able to lend a listening ear on the telephone, while others can cook meals and drive children to school.

Providing support for your loved one is even more crucial when she's undergoing interferon treatment (see Chapter 8) or getting a liver transplant (see Chapter 9).

Being a fan-club member

Your loved one may naturally feel down while living with symptoms of hepatitis C (see Chapter 4). One of the important roles of a support-team member is to have faith in your friend and to cheer him through the struggles of illness. You can be a fan-club supporter by:

- ✔ **Letting your friend or relative know she's loved and valued:** Let her know that you care and that she matters even if she has low energy or is ill. The person with hep C doesn't need to *do* anything to be loved.

- ✔ **Providing encouragement:** Encouragement is always welcome, and it's especially needed during difficult times. But remember to also provide a boost when your loved one is approaching milestones. Celebrate months or years after beginning treatment, stopping smoking, giving up alcohol, or surviving a changed job situation.

- ✔ **Joining your loved one in making healthier lifestyle changes:** See the section "Changing habits together," later in this chapter.

Here are some things that *won't* be helpful:

- ✔ **Harping on how your loved one got hep C:** However the person acquired the hep C virus, the fact is that she has it. No amount of analyzing can wish it away. Your loved one is probably upset enough about how she may have gotten it — whether from former drug use, a workplace accident, or a medical procedure. Concentrate on helping your loved one get better *now*, rather than focusing on the past.

✔ **Criticizing your loved one's decisions about treatment:** The decision of how and when to pursue different treatments is intensely personal. If you're unhappy with your spouse's choice of doctor or treatment or wish to ask them to try another approach, speak to her calmly and respectfully — once, or maybe twice. Ultimately, the final decision for treatment is up to the person with hepatitis C. The last thing your wife needs now is hurtful criticism.

✔ **Complaining about having to do all the work around the house:** Believe me, your loved one would much rather be well enough to do housework, no matter how much she hates it. To keep your own mental and physical health intact, help out only as much as you can, and no more. If you do more than you're able to, you can easily get angry or resentful, and such reactions are no help to anyone. See the section "Doing housework," later in this chapter.

Communicating with your loved one

Keeping the lines of communication open and honest can help the person with hep C. As a friend or relative, you can help by letting the person with hep C know that you're available if and when she wants to talk.

Listening is one of the most useful ways to support someone. How, when, or where your friend or relative wants to communicate is up to her, but you can let her know you're available. When your loved one starts speaking, listen without judgment. Your friend may not want any advice but may just need to vent or express thoughts and feelings.

Your loved one with hep C may have trouble communicating sensitive issues. Listen carefully when he wants to:

✔ Tell you or others about his disease or how he got it. (Deciding whom to tell and how to tell them is one of the challenges for people with hep C; see Chapter 15 for more on this topic.)

✔ Discuss frustrations and emotions about his change in health or lifestyle.

✔ Talk about fears of illness or death.

✔ Ask for help.

You might want to communicate the following things to your loved one:

✔ Your desire to help out.

✔ Your own limitations in how much you can help. Explain from the start that your time or abilities may be restricted, but you want to help nevertheless.

✔ Your own fears or sadness about the person's illness.

Different people have different ways of communicating, depending on their gender and culture. Try to be flexible, and let your relative communicate in a way that works for her.

Changing habits together

Adopting a healthier lifestyle goes along with living with hepatitis C. When people with hep C exchange unhealthy habits for life-enhancing practices, they may reduce the severity of some of their symptoms and maybe even live a longer life.

For most people, changing habits is difficult. Eating certain foods and drinks is usually the result of a lifetime of practice! Even if you know that a substance is hurting you (like cigarettes or alcohol), the attachment or even addiction to certain substances or behaviors (such as watching TV and eating junk food) can be almost impossible to conquer. Some folks with hep C may still be using drugs. Your loved one should get professional help if needed (see Chapter 12).

You can also help by changing to a healthier lifestyle yourself. Showing someone how to change by example works much better than telling the person what to do! Here are some ways to join in with your loved one to encourage the new habits:

✔ **Eat healthy meals.** Prepare them yourself, or make healthy choices when you all go out to eat. If you're watching your dining companions eat fried or sugary food, giving up unhealthy choices can be hard, especially at first. Eating healthy meals is easier if everyone in the family is eating with you.

✔ **Exercise together.** Take walks together, follow a Yoga tape, or attend a T'ai Chi class. Exercising with someone else is definitely more fun and inspiring.

✔ **Get together for meditation or religious practice.** A sense of community, shared beliefs, and purpose can lift everyone's mood.

✔ **Don't use cigarettes, drugs, or alcohol yourself** — at all or at least when you're around your friend or relative with hep C.

To get support changing your eating or exercise habits, consider going to a nutritionist (dietician), professional trainer, or mental health professional. If you or your partner are addicted to alcohol or drugs, you can both benefit from professional help (see Chapter 12). If you're giving up cigarettes, try a nicotine-replacement product, or see your doctor for other medications that might help.

Helping with healthcare

Whenever possible, the person with hep C should bring a family member or friend to all important doctor visits. Two heads are better than one at remembering what was said and asking pertinent questions. A second person can also help drive and navigate around hospitals and doctors' offices. Here are some other ways to help with your loved one's medical care:

- ✔ Help keep the hep C notebook organized. See the suggestions for keeping a hep C notebook throughout this book.
- ✔ Help fill out or file health insurance paperwork or disability benefit paperwork (see Chapter 16).
- ✔ Call the pharmacy to request refills, fill out the paperwork, and pick up prescriptions.

People with hep C who are very young, very old, or very sick especially need someone to coordinate their healthcare needs.

Living with Someone with Hep C

If you share a household with a loved one with hep C, you're in the frontline of living with the effects of the disease, but you also have the most potential to help the person cope.

Protecting yourself from infection

Hep C is spread through exposure to infected blood, so when you live in close quarters with someone who is infected, practicing good safety habits is important. However, you also need to remember not to become paranoid or fearful around the person with hep C. (See Chapter 2 for info about how hep C is transmitted and how to prevent the spread of hep C.)

Hepatitis C is *not* spread through casual contact, and members of the same household will not get the virus unless there is a blood exchange. As soon as they're old enough to understand, children in the household can be told to avoid blood from open wounds or menstruation.

Set up the household so that everyone has separate toothbrushes, toothpaste, razors, manicure scissors, pierced jewelry, and other items that may pick up small amounts of blood. If your sexual partner has hep C, see the "Being a Sexual Partner of a Person with Hep C" section, later in this chapter, and Chapter 2.

The most dangerous way to get hep C is to share any drug paraphernalia whatsoever with anyone else. (See Chapter 2 to read about transmission.)

Coordinating contacts

In an emergency or when the person with hep C simply is too fatigued to carry out normal activities, you'll need a list of people and places to contact. To prepare for those times, compose a list of important phone numbers in advance. Here are some suggestions:

- Babysitters
- Doctors and other healthcare providers
- Local hospital or clinic
- Mental health providers and social workers
- Neighbors (who may have extra keys or alarm codes)
- Religious-clergy member or spiritual adviser
- Schools
- Taxi or car service
- Trusted people to pick up your children from school
- Veterinarian or animal-care helpers
- Workplaces

Work together with your loved one to come up with a list of numbers, and make a few copies. Keep one copy in the hep C notebook and other copies in your car or briefcase. Being prepared can reduce anxiety and stress.

Doing housework

Discuss the household chores openly, and find out what your family member is able to do without compromising his health. Remember, he may be using all the energy he has just to work part-time or take his medication.

Make a detailed list of the household tasks, from cooking to cleaning to shopping. If you have children, add their needs to the list. You may need to enlist more help from family and friends, hire helpers, or live with a messier home. Another solution is to simplify your lifestyle so that taking care of the household is easier.

Keeping your home organized by reducing clutter and simplifying will help make your home easier to clean, keep you on time for appointments, and keep you up-to-date on childcare arrangements. Check out these sources:

> ✔ *Organizing For Dummies,* by Eileen Roth and Elizabeth Miles (Wiley).

> ✔ The organizational system outlined on the Web site www. flylady.net, which can be used by anyone with or without children, although it's absolutely great for families

Include your children in helping out. Even if they're young, they can help in some way, such as clearing the table or cleaning the litter box.

Watching for side effects

Hepatitis C disease and its treatment produce an array of symptoms and side effects. It's not always easy for someone living with these problems 24 hours a day, 7 days a week, to realize when there's a change, especially if it's a change in mood or behavior. You can provide a gentle mirror to your loved one and let him know if you notice anything of concern — a new symptom altogether or a symptom that has gotten worse.

By reading the chapters on symptoms of hepatitis C (Chapter 4) and interferon treatment (Chapter 8), you may be more aware of which side effects are possible.

Depression is a common and serious side effect of hepatitis C and its medical treatment. When depression is untreated, it can affect someone's entire life — from home to the workplace. Someone who is depressed is less likely to practice other healthy behaviors, such as healthy eating and drinking and exercising. More important, a depressed person is less likely to take his medication and can even be at risk of suicide.

Being a Sexual Partner of a Person with Hep C

Although rare, hepatitis C can be spread through sexual contact.

Hepatitis C is spread through blood, so avoid risky sexual practices that involve blood, or use protective barriers during these times. (See Chapter 2 for a discussion of risky behaviors associated with sexual transmission.)

You may want to get tested for hepatitis C if your sex partner is positive. If and how you change your sex practices after finding out about hep C is a personal matter to be discussed with your health-care practitioner and your partner.

A common problem with hep C infection and treatment is the effect on the libido. Taking medications, feeling fatigued or depressed, and worrying about the future have negative effects on sexual desire. I discuss these problems in Chapter 15. Find time to communicate with your loved one in other ways (such as talking, cuddling, or sitting quietly listening to music). Come up with creative ways to deal with any differences that may exist in your sexual desires (see Chapter 15 for tips on communicating).

If necessary, seek professional help from your doctor or a licensed mental health worker to deal with sexual issues.

If your partner is being treated for hepatitis C with combination peginterferon plus ribavirin — the current best treatment — you both need to practice adequate birth control methods, because the medications cause severe birth defects.

Listing Some Things You Can Do to Help

Are you looking for ways to be supportive, even if you don't live with someone with hepatitis C? Here, I list some fun or useful ways to help out. If you can't do any of these tasks yourself, then perhaps you can buy the item or service for your friend or relative.

- **Do you have a green thumb?** Most people like plants, although some folks are allergic to flowers. Cut some flowers from your garden, or buy a bunch from the florist or supermarket. If you have a garden, grow some extra veggies and supply your buddy with fresh tomatoes or greens (ideally, grown without pesticides).

- **Do you like to cook?** Try making some organic vegetable soup or a tasty casserole and storing a few batches in your friend's or relative's freezer.

✔ **Are you handy around the house?** Help your loved one install a water filtration system to get good clean water. Or make sure his fireplace is clean. Perhaps your friend or relative needs to install a grip in the bathroom to make getting in and out of the tub easier. Don't forget to get permission before making any improvements!

✔ **Do you like to sew?** If your loved one is spending lots of time in bed, consider making or buying a blanket, quilt, or special pillow with significant words or pictures.

✔ **Are you trained in the healing arts?** If you're a massage therapist, reiki practitioner, or Yoga teacher, or you're trained in another healing art or method, offer your friend some healing work. Don't take it personally if your friend isn't open to your offer at this time, however. People have different ways of relaxing and different preferences in healing techniques, and some people don't want to work with someone who knows them personally.

✔ **Do you like pampering others?** Even if you're not professionally trained, maybe you can give your friend or relative a manicure, pedicure, or hand or foot massage — if the person agrees to it. Use gentle motions and play some relaxing music to help set a peaceful mood.

Professionally trained manicurists and massage therapists know how to protect themselves from any bloodborne illness that their clients have. If you give your friend a manicure or pedicure, use your friend's or relative's instruments, because some blood could be transferred onto the manicure tools. Don't be paranoid, but take smart precautions (see the section on protecting others in Chapter 2). Make sure that any open cuts are covered while you give a massage, and avoid rubbing an open wound. Note that these precautions apply to everyone, not just people with hep C. Many people have hep C or other viruses in their blood and don't even know it, so it's best to carry out safe practices with everyone.

When offering help to others, always respect your loved one's wishes. For example, if you make soup and offer to make it again, but your loved one doesn't take you up on your offer, don't take it personally. Everyone has different tastebuds! Ask whether you can make something else or help in another way.

Helping others is about giving them what _they_ want or need, not what _you_ think they should want or need.

Part V
The Part of Tens

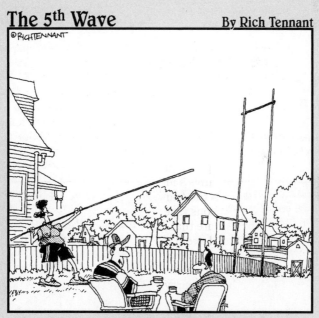

"Don't get me wrong. I think it's great that Barbara decided she wanted to exercise more after her diagnosis."

In this part . . .

*H*ere's the part of the book devoted to lists of ten, more or less. You can find advice to make traveling easier if you have hepatitis C, tips to make your sleep delicious and restful, and places to look for more info about hep C.

Chapter 20

Ten Tips for Vacationing with Hepatitis C

*T*aking a break from ordinary activities is wonderful for the mind and spirit. Having a chronic illness like hepatitis C shouldn't keep you from rest and relaxation or even excitement and adventure, if those things are more your style.

You may have no symptoms, be in the middle of drug treatment, or have some complications from cirrhosis; but whatever your situation, I bet that you can figure out some sort of break from the daily grind that'll help you recharge your batteries. Think about what you really need. Rest and naps? Good nutritious food? Peaceful communing with nature? Time with friends and family? Adventure to exotic places?

While beginning to plan for your trip, speak to your healthcare professional for recommendations tailored to fit your situation. Certain places or types of travel could have more risk of aggravating your hep C disease. Also, be realistic about your financial situation, and consult with your family.

Anticipating your needs is the way to have things go smoothly. This chapter gives you some ideas for keeping your trip safe and enjoyable.

Trying a Mini-Vacation

You may not feel ready for a long trip. You may have just been diagnosed or just started treatment for hep C. Maybe you're concerned about your energy levels or symptoms. Instead of giving up the idea of a vacation altogether, why not try a short trip near home?

You may want to make your first trip an easy half-day journey, or maybe you feel up to a full day. Use these as enjoyable trial runs for your trips farther afield. Or you may find that the mini-vacations are enough for you. Consult local newspapers for schedules of local events that interest you. Here are some ideas for getaways:

- ✓ If you live in or near a city, become a tourist again, and plan a day of sightseeing, using public transportation or walking around town. Visit a museum, see a show, or go to a sports event. You can even stay overnight in a hotel in your own city!

- ✓ If a country outing is more to your liking, walk through the woods, bike, visit a special event, or go antiquing along back roads. Try an interesting restaurant or plan a picnic dinner (weather permitting). You may want to camp or stay at a quaint bed-and-breakfast.

The point is to enjoy yourself and see how you feel. Because you're nearby, you can always return home earlier if you need to.

After your trip, note how you feel. Do you feel rejuvenated or exhausted? Is your stomach upset? Write down your experiences, particularly any problems. When you plan your next mini-vacation or a longer trip, you can use this information to make better choices.

Bringing Your Medicine

When traveling, bring along a supply of any medications you're taking that will last for the duration of your trip. But also take copies of your prescriptions — in case you run into any trouble with customs or lose your medication.

If you'll be on hep C drug treatment while traveling, speak to your doctor, preferably in the planning stages of your trip rather than a day before leaving. Your doctor should be able to give you some advice about whether she thinks that you're good to go or whether you should stay close to home in case of side effects.

Keep these considerations about your medical supplies in mind:

- ✓ When traveling with a needle or syringe, keep all medication in its original packaging. Have prescriptions handy for syringes and associated medicines.

✔ You may need to bring some type of insulated cooler to keep medications at a cold temperature. Freeze some water bottles to put in the cooler, and keep the medicines near but not touching the frozen bottle. Be sure that you don't freeze your medicine: Wrap it in a gel pack to protect it from freezing or breaking within your cooler.

Don't start a new medication just before you travel, because it can cause side effects that you may not be prepared for.

If you take herbs or vitamins, bring enough for your trip. Keep them in the original packages or bottles to avoid delays at customs or airport security (so officials don't wonder what those herbs are) or if you need to replace them.

Protecting Your Family and Others

If you have hepatitis C, you have the potential to infect others. It's especially important to remember this during travel, because your normal routine is disrupted, and you may be in closer contact with your family. Simply plan ahead:

✔ Bring your own toothbrush, toothpaste, razors, and other personal items.

✔ Keep your personal items in one or more closed plastic containers labeled with your name.

✔ Keep some adhesive bandages and other wound coverings in your wallet or purse, as well as in your luggage. Vacations and travel seem to bring about more cuts and bruises.

Practice safe sex to protect others from sexual transmission of hep C. Doing so has the added benefit of protecting you from other sexually transmitted diseases. Both male and female latex condoms are available.

Staying Healthy

You probably have a routine at home that keeps your fatigue and tummy problems away, but when you're traveling, everything is different. For this reason, many people are scared of travel. But you can practice good self-care even when you're vacationing:

✔ **Make sure to get enough rest.** Don't go to bed late if you have to wake up early. Take as many naps as you want. This is a vacation, remember?

✔ **Don't overdo it.** Most folks get excited when they're discovering a new place, so they want to see and do everything. Avoid that temptation. Enjoy one garden, one museum (or even one room in a museum), or one city rather than ten gardens in a morning, five museums in a day, or ten cities in a week. The quality of your experience matters more than the quantity, especially when overdoing it may put you flat on your back in exhaustion.

✔ **Drink plenty of water.** Take water bottles with you everywhere. They'll keep you hydrated and help with just about everything (how's that for a superscientific explanation?).

✔ **Eat with care.** Temptations abound to eat junk food or rich exotic food. If you have problems with your digestion, consider these tips:

- Think twice before indulging in fried fatty food.

- Bring healthy snacks that you know agree with you.

- Go to restaurants that offer you choices that usually don't upset your stomach.

- Plan ahead. If you know that you need to eat every three hours, and you'll be on the road, bring snacks for the car, or plan to stop at a suitable restaurant.

✔ **Watch out for the sun and humidity.** Your medications may make you more sensitive to the sun. Use sunscreen, sunglasses, a hat, and long-sleeved, light-colored clothing to protect you from the sun. Better yet, take a siesta when the sun is high in the sky.

For your own safety, I recommend getting the hepatitis A and hepatitis B vaccines, if you're not already immune to these viruses (determined by testing your blood). As described in Chapter 2, getting another type of hepatitis virus could lead to more serious illness. Even if you never leave the United States, these vaccinations are recommended.

Flying with Ease

No, I can't explain how to flap your wings, but I can tell you how to make flying in a plane more pleasant.

✔ Wear comfortable clothing.

✔ Reduce stress by giving yourself plenty of time to get to the airport.

✔ Call your airline in advance to see whether you have choices in food plans, such as fruit or vegetarian meals.

✔ Bring bottled water and healthy snacks. If you have to sit in the airport during a flight delay, airport food options may not be the healthiest ones.

✔ If you have trouble walking, ask the airline for help getting to your gate. The airlines will drive you through the airport or provide a wheelchair.

✔ Bring sanitary wipes or a liquid disinfectant with you. Thousands of passengers travel on airplanes and pass through airports every day, so you risk catching some airborne illness. Cleaning your hands frequently may prevent you from catching some germs.

Choosing Foreign Travel Destinations

The farther you go from home and the less developed the destination country is, the more risk you take if things go awry. In developing countries, funds and the government infrastructure are not in place to reliably protect the water supplies, food sources, or blood supply. Tropical countries have diseases like malaria and yellow fever, which are transmitted through mosquito bites. The water, food, and even the blood supply can be contaminated with infectious agents.

When traveling within the United States and Canada or to Japan, Australia, New Zealand, and Western Europe, your risks are much less.

Vaccination against infectious diseases is required for travel to many developing countries. When traveling to developing countries, find out which vaccines or prevention medicines you should take. Also, if you're traveling to more than one country, check out how that affects your vaccination requirements. Here are a few sources:

✔ **U.S. Centers for Disease Control:** The travel section of the U.S. Centers for Disease Control and Prevention Web site, www.cdc.gov, has links for travel clinics in each state as well as a wealth of information on travel destinations.

✔ **International Society of Travel Medicine:** Check out www.istm.org, which lists travel clinics all over the world (including the United States and Canada).

These travel clinics offer pretrip advising and vaccination as well as post-travel medical consultation.

If you are on any type of interferon treatment or are taking immuno-suppressive medication after a liver transplant, you must consult your doctor before your trip. These medications affect your immune system, and you may be advised to take extra care or even avoid foreign travel, which may expose you to dangerous infections.

Steering Clear of Travelers' Diarrhea

Travel to foreign countries with unprotected water supplies means that you or anyone in your family may get an infection that causes travelers' diarrhea. If you have liver problems, you may be more sensitive to such an infection.

Your doctor may give you antibiotics to bring along in case you get sick. Speak to your healthcare provider, who will properly advise you on prevention strategies.

Here are tips for preventing travelers' diarrhea through safe eating and drinking practices:

- ✔ Eat food that has been cooked thoroughly, is still hot, and hasn't been sitting around unheated for a long period of time.

- ✔ Avoid uncooked food, except fruits and vegetables that you peel or shell yourself.

- ✔ Avoid dishes containing raw or undercooked eggs.

- ✔ Don't buy food from street vendors.

- ✔ Drink only beverages that come from bottles or cans or that have been boiled.

- ✔ Use bottled (or boiled) water for brushing your teeth.

- ✔ Avoid ice unless you know it has been made from purified water.

Concerning Mosquito-Borne Infections

Travelers must provide vaccination papers for yellow fever and malaria when traveling to many tropical locales, and these diseases can present special complications for folks with hepatitis C. Check with your doctor, travel agent, a travel guide, or the www.cdc.gov Web site to see whether either of these infections is a problem where you're traveling:

✔ **Yellow fever:** Yellow fever is a virus transmitted through mosquitoes and can be prevented by immunization. The vaccination against yellow fever uses a live vaccine.

✔ **Malaria:** This parasite is transmitted through another type of mosquito (not the mosquito that spreads yellow fever). You need to take preventive antimalaria medications (called *prophylactic medication*), but some of these can cause damage to your liver. Your doctor will advise you on which medications to take.

Avoiding mosquito bites is important in the tropics, where you may encounter malaria or yellow fever. (It's also a good idea to avoid being bitten in the United States, where mosquitoes can transmit West Nile virus.) Ways to avoid being bitten include

✔ Try to stay inside when insects are biting (usually at night, but this differs among different types of insects). Make sure that you have adequate protection when sleeping: good screens on windows, netting over your bed, or insect-repellent coils.

✔ If you go outside when insects are biting, wear long-sleeved clothing, and tuck your shirt in. You might need to use an insect repellent. The most-used and -tested bug spray contains DEET, which repels mosquitoes, ticks, and other bugs. Read and follow the labels of any insect repellents you use. DEET and other pesticides are toxins and should be used with extreme caution, washed off when you're inside, and avoided if possible.

Getting Medical Care Abroad

Prepare for the unexpected. During travel to foreign countries, you could have an accident or medical emergency and need urgent medical care. Discuss with your doctor or travel specialist bringing certain medications for self-treatment in case you become ill.

Find out in advance what your health insurance will cover when you are overseas. Medicare, for example, doesn't cover hospital or medical costs outside the United States. If your policy provides coverage in foreign countries, get copies of any bills or receipts, and carry an insurance policy card and claim forms with you. Try to obtain travel insurance that provides assistance if you get ill or have a medical emergency. You may have to pay in advance and get reimbursed later.

In developing countries, you're at risk if you require medical procedures that use reused needles or blood transfusions. The blood supply may be contaminated with HIV, hepatitis B, or hepatitis C (you can get other genotypes on top of your own infection).

Avoiding Dangerous Practices

You can have fun while traveling! But avoid the temptation to take risks while on vacation or in foreign countries. I'm assuming you've taken my advice, given throughout this book, to avoid alcohol and injecting drugs altogether. Certainly, don't drink or use drugs in a foreign country! You need to keep your wits about you.

Because of less sanitary conditions in developing countries, leave the tattoos and piercings for when you get home. You risk catching HIV or other infections from unsterilized equipment. Even with a clean needle, the ink from the tattoo pot could be reused, and you could exchange a virus with the last client or the next one.

Having unprotected sex at any time is risky. Protect yourself from HIV, hepatitis B, or other sexually transmitted diseases by using a latex male condom or a female condom. You should also protect others from your hepatitis C virus.

Swimming in natural bodies of water can be a potential risk, because the water may be polluted with sewage. Even swimming pools with chlorine may have some contamination. Don't swallow any water, and avoid entering the water if you have unprotected cuts or wounds.

Chapter 21

Ten Tips for Sleeping Well with Hepatitis C

In This Chapter

▶ Getting enough exercise and fresh air

▶ Creating comfortable sleeping conditions

▶ Using scents or tapes to relax

*G*etting a good night's sleep is important for everyone. You need your sleep to rejuvenate your body, mind, and emotions. For folks facing an illness like hepatitis C, you can see why this nightly revitalization is even more important.

But the twist is that the physical and emotional stresses and complications that folks with hep C face can wreak havoc with the nighttime nap. Stress, anxiety, night sweats, hep C medications, aches and pains, depression, or other illnesses can all contribute to insomnia: difficulty falling asleep, difficulty remaining asleep, or waking up too early.

Don't take any over-the-counter sleeping remedies unless they're recommended by a healthcare practitioner who's knowledgeable about liver disease. Some products contain substances that could hurt your liver (see Chapter 12 for info on toxic substances).

In this chapter, I give you some safe self-help tips to help you get a good night's sleep. If you find that you still have trouble sleeping after following these tips, discuss the problem with your doctor, who can recommend or prescribe sleeping remedies or medications.

Get Exercise and Country Air

When you lie down to sleep, make sure that your body is good and tired and ready for bed by moving it during the day (see Chapter 13 for suggestions on exercise and movement). But don't exercise for a few hours right before bedtime, because doing so can keep you awake.

You know that old saying about country air's giving you a good appetite and a good night's sleep? It's worth a try. Get fresh air by using deep-breathing techniques (see Chapter 13), getting some outdoor exercise during the day, opening your windows at night, or using an air purifier if you live in a polluted environment.

Eat and Drink for Sleepy Times

By avoiding stimulants and increasing foods that contribute to good sleep, you can help your body start yawning. Consider this advice:

- ✔ Try to eliminate caffeine from your diet or at least limit the amount and have it only early in the day. Coffee, tea, sodas, and chocolate may have caffeine.

- ✔ Stop smoking. Nicotine (in cigarettes) is a stimulant.

- ✔ Make sure that your diet includes enough carbohydrates, calcium, and magnesium (which help you sleep). Tryptophan, an amino acid in milk, also helps induce sleep, so try drinking a glass of cold milk (or a mug of hot milk) near bedtime.

- ✔ Avoid eating large meals late at night. Eat an early dinner, and make lunch your biggest meal of the day.

Take Naps

Naps are the holy grail for some people with hep C. If you're dealing with fatigue and low energy, you may absolutely need your naps. On the other hand, some people think that naps can lead to lack of sleepiness at night. Try to have your naps earlier in the day, and don't nap for hours and hours if you find that doing so disturbs your nighttime sleep.

Sleep on a Schedule

Establish a regular schedule for going to bed and waking up each day. Prepare for your "sleep date" by getting ready in advance and starting to relax. At the set time, turn off the lights. Set your alarm to wake you at a preset time in the morning. For some people, a routine helps them get their needed sleep.

Create a Bedroom for Sleeping

People don't live in magazines, so you may not always be able to keep your bedroom clean, clutter-free, and cozy. But having a calm and comfy bedroom is important if you're having trouble sleeping:

- ✔ Make sure that your bedding is clean and comfortable. Don't use blankets that are too heavy, and make sure your pillows support your neck.

- ✔ Keep the temperature just right. If you need a cooler room, lower the heat or use air conditioning. If you're feeling too cold, use a hot-water bottle.

- ✔ Use your bed for sleep and sex, and nothing else. If you watch TV or read, do it somewhere else.

- ✔ Create a quiet, dark environment for sleeping.

Relax before Bed

Set your body up for delicious sleep by setting the stage with relaxation. Before you go to bed, take a bath, read a relaxing book (not an exiting book that'll keep you up all night finishing it), or meditate or do progressive relaxation (see Chapter 13). Avoid stimulating television, heated conversations, or exercise just before bedtime; these activities may keep you awake.

Try Aromatherapy

Certain scents, such as lavender, neroli, rose, sandalwood, and chamomile, may help you to relax into a blissful sleep. Smelling something pleasant is a soothing distraction from what keeps you from falling asleep.

Try essential (pure) oils or fragrance oils that you can find in health food stores. To spread (diffuse) the scent around your room, you can use a store-bought diffuser or try one of these tips:

- ✔ Add a couple of drops of oil to a cotton ball or a mug of hot water on your nightstand.

- ✔ Fill a spray bottle with purified or distilled water and a few drops of scent, and spray your pillow before you go to bed.

- ✔ Use the oils (sparingly) in a bedtime bath, or use a specially made aromatherapy pillow (with lavender flowers, for example).

You can also try rubbing a body lotion/oil with your favorite scent on your hands and arms before you go to sleep.

A little scent can go a long way. Start with a little bit; if you use too much, it can disturb you or your sleeping partner.

Listen to Tapes

During the period while you're getting ready to go to sleep or after you turn off the lights, try listening to some relaxing music or tapes. When you're focused on the music, sounds, or words on the tape, your mind won't be focused on worries. Depending on what tapes you choose to listen to, you can be diverted, amused, or uplifted.

Have you ever found yourself being soothed or sleepy while someone spoke to you? Although the speaker may not appreciate that you're drifting off while he speaks his heart out, the spoken word can sometimes be like a lullaby. I use this method when my mind is too busy to let me sleep.

Wear Comfortable Bedclothes

After you set the stage for sleep with a comfy bed; cool, fresh air; nice aromatherapy scent; clean light sheets; and a dark, quiet room, it's time to think about what you wear to bed. Wear clothing that isn't tight fitting so that you can move your body with ease. Also try wearing cotton clothing if you have night sweats, which can happen with hepatitis C.

Waking Up Too Early

Ah, you've fallen asleep at last. But then you find yourself awake while it's still pitch-black outside, nowhere near dawn. If you awaken and can't get back to sleep, don't spend too much time tossing and turning. You can stay in bed and listen to a relaxation tape or do some relaxation exercises. Or get out of bed and read a book. Ideally, you'll soon be able to return to sweet dreams.

Whether you can't get to sleep in the first place or get back to sleep in the middle of the night, don't lie in bed worrying about not getting enough sleep. You'll only become more anxious, which will just prevent you from being able to fall asleep!

Chapter 22

Ten-Plus Web Sites and Resources for Hep C

*I*f you want to do further research about hepatitis C, a wealth of information is out there to help you find out about a new clinical trial, look up a drug you're taking, find other people with hepatitis C, or just look around to feel more connected.

As you probably know, the Internet is a rich source of information on these topics. If you do a Web search on the phrase "hepatitis C," you'll get more than 1 million hits, or possible links to hepatitis C. But who has the time to investigate all of these sites?

In this chapter, I help you narrow down your search for information by listing some of the heavy hitters — the sites you may need most or don't want to miss. These sites also direct you, through Web links, to other great sources of information. Happy surfing!

 Because Web sites frequently rearrange their pages, if you go to a site and don't find the link, go to the home page for that site, and navigate on the site map or do a search on your topic of interest.

Centers for Disease Control and Prevention (CDC)

The Centers for Disease Control and Prevention (CDC) has information in English and Spanish on testing, prevention, and education about hepatitis C, as well as other hepatitis viruses. This site gives you the basic information on transmission and prevention, and has links to other government sites for discussion of treatment.

Here's the contact info: Centers for Disease Control and Prevention, 1600 Clifton Rd., Atlanta, GA 30333; phone 404-639-3311, public inquiries 404-639-3534 and 800-311-3435; Web site www.cdc.gov/ncidod/diseases/hepatitis/c.

MedlinePlus Health Information

MedlinePlus is an all-encompassing online service of the U.S. National Library of Medicine and National Institutes of Health. You can find a medical encyclopedia, information on drugs, news articles, and more by using the search engine. Go to www.medline plus.gov or www.medlineplus.gov/Spanish for the Spanish version.

You can find a wealth of information about hepatitis C, different manifestations of the illness (such as cirrhosis or depression), tests and what they mean, and different drugs and their side effects. In other words, you can find information on most aspects of the disease and treatment for hepatitis C. Start your search by entering "hepatitis C" or "cirrhosis." In addition to the encyclopedia, the site includes links to many U.S. medical sites.

Veterans Affairs National Hepatitis C Program

The Department of Veterans Affairs sponsors this Web site, www.hepatitis.va.gov, which provides a huge amount of information about viral hepatitis for veterans, healthcare providers inside and outside the VA system, and the general public. You can find everything from an art gallery of work made by veterans with hepatitis C to information on starting a support group.

Hepatitis C Advocate

The HCV Advocate (www.hcvadvocate.org) is a comprehensive source of information about hepatitis C on the Web. It offers simply written fact sheets (in English and Spanish), educational information in additional languages from Chinese to Russian to French, news updates, and a series of expert articles on different medical topics related to hepatitis C. The site includes a monthly newsletter with thoughtful commentaries on the latest hep C medical news and events. The Hepatitis C Support Project (HCSP), a registered non-profit organization founded in 1997 by Alan Franciscus.

American Liver Foundation

The American Liver Foundation (ALF) is a national nonprofit organization dedicated to research, education, and advocacy for the prevention and treatment of liver disease, including hepatitis C. The ALF produces patient materials in English and Spanish, provides information on support groups, and has different chapters all over the country. Find your chapter so you can get involved with hepatitis C events in your area.

Here's how to contact them: American Liver Foundation, 75 Maiden Lane, Suite 603, New York, NY 10038; phone 800-GO-LIVER (800-465-4837) or 888-443-7222; e-mail info@liverfoundation.org; Web site www.liverfoundation.org.

Hepatitis C Choices

The Hepatitis C Caring Ambassadors Program has produced an online manual that describes different healthcare choices (including Western, ayurvedic, homeopathic, naturopathic, and traditional Chinese medicine). Check it out at www.hepcchallenge.org/manual.

The Hepatitis C Association

The Hepatitis C Association aims to provide support and education to people concerned with hepatitis C. You can contact them at 866-437-4377. They have a message board called "Hepatitis C Association Voices" that you can access at www.hepcassoc.org.

Hepatitis Neighborhood

This informational site (www.hepatitisneighborhood.com) is run by Priority Healthcare Corporation and has educational and support information as well as online chats. You must sign up, but it's free.

Hep C Connection

Based in Denver, Colorado, Hep C Connection (www.hepc-connection.org) promotes support and education for people with hep C. The group has a quarterly newsletter, info on support groups, and a hep C hotline (800-522-HEPC).

HIV and Hepatitis

This Web site (www.hivandhepatitis.com) has loads of research information on hepatitis C as well as on hepatitis C and HIV co-infection. You can find regularly updated articles as well a section called "The Doctor Is In" where you can submit questions on treatment.

Hepatitis Foundation International

Hepatitis Foundation International provides education, support and doctor referrals for all types of hepatitis.

Contact this organization at Hepatitis Foundation International, 504 Blick Drive, Silver Spring, MD 20904-2901; phone 800-891-0707 (to speak to a counselor or obtain information); Web site www.hepfi.org.

World Health Organization (WHO)

A branch of the United Nations, the World Health Organization (WHO) is run by 192 member states via the World Health Assembly. It offers information on dozens of health topics, including figures on the worldwide prevalence of hepatitis C. You can find branches of the WHO all over the world. If you want to read about hepatitis C in Egypt, this is the place. The Web site is www.who.int.

Sources Outside the United States

This section provides some Web-based information from other English-speaking countries. Although some information is specific for a particular location, much of it is applicable to everyone.

Australia

The Australia Hepatitis Council provides an extensive information resource on hepatitis at its Web site, www.hepatitis australia.com.

The Hepatitis C Council of New South Wales (www.hepatitisc. org.au) invites you to check out its fact sheets, educational articles, and online magazine, *Hep C Review,* which has great regional contact information for everyone concerned with hepatitis C, as well as a review of all things related to hepatitis C.

Canada

The Canadian Liver Foundation has information about hep C in English and French at its Web site, www.liver.ca. It also has links to regional chapters throughout Canada.

If you're Canadian with hep C, the Health Canada site (www. phac-aspc.gc.ca/hepc/hepatitis_c) wants to hear from you about your experiences in obtaining hep C healthcare services. And the Hepatitis C Society of Canada (www.hepatitiscsociety. com) has links to support throughout the country.

United Kingdom

The Hepatitis C Trust (www.hepcuk.info) in the United Kingdom provides an online resource that gives clear information on hepatitis C issues specific to the United Kingdom, as well as general information on living with hepatitis C.

The British Liver Trust (www.britishlivertrust.org.uk) is a charity that covers all liver diseases, including hepatitis C. You can get some information translated into Urdu, Bengali, and Hindi. You can also find information on U.K. transplant units and support for nurses who work with hepatitis C.

Drug Companies

The companies that make drugs for hepatitis C provide patient support by providing information, helping you get through the treatment with support programs, and giving financial support if you can't afford treatment. I list the pharmaceutical companies that produce peginterferon and ribavirin, the treatment for hep C patients:

✔ **Schering-Plough:** These folks produce Peg-Intron (peginterferon alfa-2b) and Rebetol (ribavirin). For information about financial assistance for eligible patients through the Commitment to Care Program, call 800-521-7157 or visit www.hepatitisinnovations.com (click "Resources" in the Quick Links drop-down list).

For emotional support while you're taking the medication, turn to the Be In Charge Program and Readipen assistance. Call 888-HEP-2608 (437-2608) or visit www.beincharge.com.

✔ **Hoffmann-La Roche:** This company makes Pegasys (Peginterferon alfa-2a) and Copegus (ribavirin).

For financial help, call the Pegasys reimbursement hotline and patient-assistance program at 800-387-1258. If you meet certain criteria, the drug therapy is shipped to your healthcare provider's office at no charge.

For the education and support program, call 877-PEGASYS (877-734-2797) to reach the Pegassist program, or get online at www.pegassist.com.

If you're interested in the drug Infergen, go to www.infergen.com, and click the "Patients" tab.

Index

• Q •

BUSINESS, CAREERS & PERSONAL FINANCE

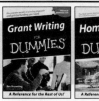

0-7645-5307-0   0-7645-5331-3 *†

Also available:

✔Accounting For Dummies †
0-7645-5314-3
✔Business Plans Kit For Dummies †
0-7645-5365-8
✔Cover Letters For Dummies
0-7645-5224-4
✔Frugal Living For Dummies
0-7645-5403-4
✔Leadership For Dummies
0-7645-5176-0
✔Managing For Dummies
0-7645-1771-6

✔Marketing For Dummies
0-7645-5600-2
✔Personal Finance For Dummies *
0-7645-2590-5
✔Project Management
For Dummies
0-7645-5283-X
✔Resumes For Dummies †
0-7645-5471-9
✔Selling For Dummies
0-7645-5363-1
✔Small Business Kit For Dummies *†
0-7645-5093-4

HOME & BUSINESS COMPUTER BASICS

0-7645-4074-2   0-7645-3758-X

Also available:

✔ACT! 6 For Dummies
0-7645-2645-6
✔iLife '04 All-in-One Desk Reference
For Dummies
0-7645-7347-0
✔iPAQ For Dummies
0-7645-6769-1
✔Mac OS X Panther Timesaving
Techniques For Dummies
0-7645-5812-9
✔Macs For Dummies
0-7645-5656-8
✔Microsoft Money 2004 For Dummies
0-7645-4195-1

✔Office 2003 All-in-One Desk
Reference For Dummies
0-7645-3883-7
✔Outlook 2003 For Dummies
0-7645-3759-8
✔PCs For Dummies
0-7645-4074-2
✔TiVo For Dummies
0-7645-6923-6
✔Upgrading and Fixing PCs
For Dummies
0-7645-1665-5
✔Windows XP Timesaving
Techniques For Dummies
0-7645-3748-2

FOOD, HOME, GARDEN, HOBBIES, MUSIC & PETS

0-7645-5295-3   0-7645-5232-5

Also available:

✔Bass Guitar For Dummies
0-7645-2487-9
✔Diabetes Cookbook For Dummies
0-7645-5230-9
✔Gardening For Dummies *
0-7645-5130-2
✔Guitar For Dummies
0-7645-5106-X
✔Holiday Decorating For Dummies
0-7645-2570-0
✔Home Improvement All-in-One
For Dummies
0-7645-5680-0

✔Knitting For Dummies
0-7645-5395-X
✔Piano For Dummies
0-7645-5105-1
✔Puppies For Dummies
0-7645-5255-4
✔Scrapbooking For Dummies
0-7645-7208-3
✔Senior Dogs For Dummies
0-7645-5818-8
✔Singing For Dummies
0-7645-2475-5
✔30-Minute Meals For Dummies
0-7645-2589-1

INTERNET & DIGITAL MEDIA

0-7645-1664-7   0-7645-6924-4

Also available:

✔2005 Online Shopping Directory
For Dummies
0-7645-7495-7
✔CD & DVD Recording For Dummies
0-7645-5956-7
✔eBay For Dummies
0-7645-5654-1
✔Fighting Spam For Dummies
0-7645-5965-6
✔Genealogy Online For Dummies
0-7645-5964-8
✔Google For Dummies
0-7645-4420-9

✔Home Recording For Musicians
For Dummies
0-7645-1634-5
✔The Internet For Dummies
0-7645-4173-0
✔iPod & iTunes For Dummies
0-7645-7772-7
✔Preventing Identity Theft
For Dummies
0-7645-7336-5
✔Pro Tools All-in-One Desk
Reference For Dummies
0-7645-5714-9
✔Roxio Easy Media Creator
For Dummies
0-7645-7131-1

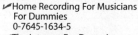

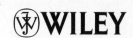

SPORTS, FITNESS, PARENTING, RELIGION & SPIRITUALITY

0-7645-5146-9

0-7645-5418-2

Also available:

- Adoption For Dummies
  0-7645-5488-3
- Basketball For Dummies
  0-7645-5248-1
- The Bible For Dummies
  0-7645-5296-1
- Buddhism For Dummies
  0-7645-5359-3
- Catholicism For Dummies
  0-7645-5391-7
- Hockey For Dummies
  0-7645-5228-7

- Judaism For Dummies
  0-7645-5299-6
- Martial Arts For Dummies
  0-7645-5358-5
- Pilates For Dummies
  0-7645-5397-6
- Religion For Dummies
  0-7645-5264-3
- Teaching Kids to Read
  For Dummies
  0-7645-4043-2
- Weight Training For Dummies
  0-7645-5168-X
- Yoga For Dummies
  0-7645-5117-5

TRAVEL

0-7645-5438-7

0-7645-5453-0

Also available:

- Alaska For Dummies
  0-7645-1761-9
- Arizona For Dummies
  0-7645-6938-4
- Cancún and the Yucatán
  For Dummies
  0-7645-2437-2
- Cruise Vacations For Dummies
  0-7645-6941-4
- Europe For Dummies
  0-7645-5456-5
- Ireland For Dummies
  0-7645-5455-7

- Las Vegas For Dummies
  0-7645-5448-4
- London For Dummies
  0-7645-4277-X
- New York City For Dummies
  0-7645-6945-7
- Paris For Dummies
  0-7645-5494-8
- RV Vacations For Dummies
  0-7645-5443-3
- Walt Disney World & Orlando
  For Dummies
  0-7645-6943-0

GRAPHICS, DESIGN & WEB DEVELOPMENT

0-7645-4345-8

0-7645-5589-8

Also available:

- Adobe Acrobat 6 PDF
  For Dummies
  0-7645-3760-1
- Building a Web Site For Dummies
  0-7645-7144-3
- Dreamweaver MX 2004
  For Dummies
  0-7645-4342-3
- FrontPage 2003 For Dummies
  0-7645-3882-9
- HTML 4 For Dummies
  0-7645-1995-6
- Illustrator cs For Dummies
  0-7645-4084-X

- Macromedia Flash MX 2004
  For Dummies
  0-7645-4358-X
- Photoshop 7 All-in-One Desk
  Reference For Dummies
  0-7645-1667-1
- Photoshop cs Timesaving
  Techniques For Dummies
  0-7645-6782-9
- PHP 5 For Dummies
  0-7645-4166-8
- PowerPoint 2003 For Dummies
  0-7645-3908-6
- QuarkXPress 6 For Dummies
  0-7645-2593-X

NETWORKING, SECURITY, PROGRAMMING & DATABASES

0-7645-6852-3

0-7645-5784-X

Also available:

- A+ Certification For Dummies
  0-7645-4187-0
- Access 2003 All-in-One Desk
  Reference For Dummies
  0-7645-3988-4
- Beginning Programming
  For Dummies
  0-7645-4997-9
- C For Dummies
  0-7645-7068-4
- Firewalls For Dummies
  0-7645-4048-3
- Home Networking For Dummies
  0-7645-42796

- Network Security For Dummies
  0-7645-1679-5
- Networking For Dummies
  0-7645-1677-9
- TCP/IP For Dummies
  0-7645-1760-0
- VBA For Dummies
  0-7645-3989-2
- Wireless All In-One Desk Reference
  For Dummies
  0-7645-7496-5
- Wireless Home Networking
  For Dummies
  0-7645-3910-8